LET BURN

LET BURN

The Making and Breaking of a Firefighter/Paramedic

Rachel K. Wentz

Michigan State University Press
East Lansing

∞ The paper used in this publication meets the minimum requirements of ANSI/NISO Z39.48-1992 (R 1997) (Permanence of Paper).

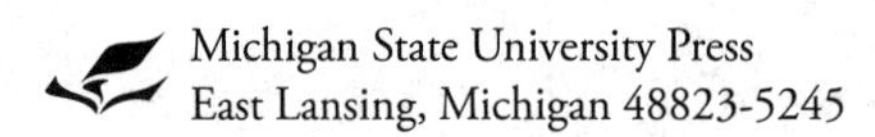
Michigan State University Press
East Lansing, Michigan 48823-5245

Printed and bound in the United States of America.

19 18 17 16 15 14 13   1 2 3 4 5 6 7 8 9 10

LIBRARY OF CONGRESS CATALOGING-IN-PUBLICATION DATA

Wentz, Rachel K.
Let burn : the making and breaking of a firefighter/paramedic / Rachel K. Wentz.
pages cm
ISBN 978-1-61186-071-9 (pbk. : alk. paper)—ISBN 978-1-60917-357-9 (ebook)
1. Wentz, R. K. 2. Women fire fighters—Florida—Biography. 3. Allied health personnel—Florida—Biography. 4. Orlando (Fla.). Fire Dept. I. Title.

TH9118.W46A3 2013
616.02'5092—dc23   [B]   2012029290

Book design by Scribe Inc. (www.scribenet.com)
Cover design by Erin Kirk New
Cover photo © iStockphoto.com

green press INITIATIVE Michigan State University Press is a member of the Green Press Initiative and is committed to developing and encouraging ecologically responsible publishing practices. For more information about the Green Press Initiative and the use of recycled paper in book publishing, please visit www.greenpressinitiative.org.

Visit Michigan State University Press at www.msupress.org

To John

Whose pride and lack of moral courage changed my life.

Let Burn—a policy of the U.S. Forestry Service
that allows wildfires to burn unchecked.
Although highly destructive, the fires leave behind
rejuvenated soils, a landscape cleared of underbrush,
and an environment ripe for new growth.

CONTENTS

INTRODUCTION

EACH OF US IS THE SUM OF OUR EXPERIENCES. OUR PERSONALITIES are carved out by events in our lives, just as water carves out a canyon. Torrents tear away the walls of our psyche, leaving voids where solid ground once stood. Steady currents strip away our interior, shaping us in ways that can only be seen later, on reflection. Painful memories become smooth, like a stone in a river, their edges worn away over time.

For thirteen years I worked as a firefighter/paramedic, primarily for the Orlando Fire Department (OFD). I began my career working for a small department just outside of Orlando. I also worked for an ambulance service in Orlando and later, for a short time, with a county agency north of Nashville, Tennessee. I spent eleven years with OFD, becoming only the third woman in the history of the department to achieve the rank of lieutenant.

These settings provided an array of perspectives. Working on an ambulance sharpened my skills as a medic. The small, rural service in Tennessee exposed me to challenges of a system where backup is nonexistent. My career with OFD placed me among highly trained individuals in a large metropolitan area. There, I honed my skills, not only as an emergency medical services (EMS) provider, but as a future officer. Through education, training, and promotional exams, I prepared myself for a leadership position within the department. I learned to be adaptive and flexible under changing circumstances, valuable lessons that would help me when I suddenly found my career cut short.

As a firefighter and medic, I saw things I never could have imagined—traumatic injury, burns, cardiac arrest, and the violence people inflict on each other. And I took on challenges I never could have anticipated in my desire to succeed. But within a moment, all that I had achieved was gone. A single decision meant the end of my accomplishments, my future as an officer, and my career.

This book recounts the incredible experiences of becoming and working as a firefighter-paramedic and the events that led to the end of my career with the Orlando Fire Department. It was hard to leave the field of EMS. You grow accustomed to the daily dose of adrenaline, and when it's gone, you're left with a nagging sense of restlessness. I left the field of EMS and completed a PhD in anthropology. I hoped the intellectual challenge would replace the physical and emotional challenges of my previous occupation. In many ways it did. In other ways, I still feel the pull of a field that shapes you as an individual. So I maintain my paramedic license out of a sense of remembrance and loss, the remembrance of being a young rookie beginning a new career and the loss of knowing those days are part of an unalterable past.

The field of EMS changed me. It carved out a personality I never knew existed, one of aggression, intensity, and determination. The physical demands of firefighting, combined with the emotional challenges of dealing with the sick and the dead, produce profound changes in an individual. It is a rare opportunity to be tested in such a way.

Within these pages, I have tried to re-create my experiences in the field. The book is divided into four parts. The first recounts my experiences upon entering the field and what it was like to acclimate to the world of firefighting and EMS. These experiences shaped me as a professional. The second part recounts my work as a firefighter-paramedic, primarily with the Orlando Fire Department, where I spent the majority of my career on some of the busiest trucks in the city. The third part provides an overview of my rise up the chain of command at OFD and the education and experience that went into that process. The fourth recounts the events that led to the end of my career. It has taken me over a decade to gain the perspective needed to put these events down on paper, to formulate the necessary detachment that comes with time and introspection.

These memories invoke pleasure and pain, but also a sense of longing: longing for the excitement I felt upon entering the field, for the camaraderie of the fire department, and for a career that was cut short. But the end of my career meant the start of a new one. It forced me into the intellectual arena of a doctoral program, and I took with me the hard-earned lessons of EMS. These lessons instilled in me a perspective few jobs can. They have given me an appreciation for the brevity of our existence and the frailty of the human body where, within a split second, all that you are and all that you have can be ripped from you. These lessons are priceless.

PART ONE

INTO THE FIELD

GETTING STARTED

I never intended to become a firefighter; I knew nothing of the profession. My introduction to the fire service was the result of my interest in medicine. I was attending the University of Central Florida, studying my first love, anthropology. But I knew that a future in anthropology meant years of study and I was young and impatient. I wanted the freedom that came with financial independence from my parents, which meant settling on a career in which I could be trained and educated within a reasonable time frame. The most important thing to me was a job that was challenging and pushed me to excel; one that would incorporate my interest in medicine with the ability to assist those in need. My father, a navy captain and chaplain, always said that if I had a job in which I helped people, I would always have a reason to get up in the morning.

So I spent a rainy afternoon in the university's library, scanning books on career opportunities and training programs. Sitting among the narrow shelves, I focused on the professions I found interesting. The job of a paramedic had always intrigued me. What could be more purposeful than assisting people in emergency situations, when they need help the most?

I grew up watching the show *Emergency* and found the profession fascinating. Paramedics are faced with different types of emergencies each shift—variety well suited to my short attention span. The fact that it involved medicine also drew me. At a very early age, I developed a fascination with the human body, especially the skeleton. I was amazed by the complex anatomical and physiological systems that make up our bodies—the thousands of chemical reactions that take place each second in order to sustain life. Growing up the daughter of a naval officer, I relished the times when my mother would usher me and my siblings into the base hospital for our vaccinations prior to traveling overseas. To me, hospitals were encapsulated worlds of human drama. I would wander the halls while awaiting our appointment, the cool smell of disinfectant stinging my nostrils. I watched the staff rush from room to room, wondering what was happening to the people inside. I was drawn to the field of medicine from the start.

I found a book describing the education and training involved in becoming a paramedic and set to work. The local community college offered a program and I quickly applied, just making the deadline for new applicants. The first step in the process was becoming an emergency medical technician (EMT); the training consisted of a semester of coursework followed by a semester of fieldwork. EMTs are trained in basic lifesaving procedures, including bandaging, splinting, and cardiopulmonary resuscitation (CPR). But I wanted more. I wanted to be able to administer medications, start intravenous (IV) lines, and perform advanced medical procedures. So I set my sights on completing the EMT program and going straight into paramedic school. My paramedic training would consist of two semesters of coursework, sitting for the state exam, and a "provisional" period of fieldwork during which I would complete an extensive checklist of skills before being allowed to practice on my own. The fieldwork began.

DOWN AND OUT

THE ROOTS OF OUR NATION'S EMERGENCY MEDICAL SERVICES (EMS) actually began in Europe during Napoleon's military campaigns of the early 1800s. His physician, Dominique-Jean Larrey, was one of the first to note that expedient ground transport of injured soldiers to field hospitals could improve survival rates. These practices were later incorporated into American military campaigns. During World War I, the first field "medics" accompanied ground soldiers onto the battlefield. By World War II, medics were cross-trained as soldiers, and the era of the combat medic was born. During the Korean and Vietnam conflicts, helicopters became the most expedient means of transporting the injured. This quick transport, combined with more sophisticated equipment and field hospitals, vastly improved survival rates among combat personnel. Many of these groundbreaking techniques and practices evolved into today's EMS systems, with expedient and effective transport and treatment of the injured being the primary objective of prehospital care.

EMT and paramedic programs in the United States prepare future EMS providers through a combination of course curriculum and field training. In the classroom, they learn the fundamentals of anatomy and physiology, a range of treatment procedures used in the field, and the skills to administer these treatments. Fieldwork is where they practice their skills on live patients under the supervision of experienced professionals, either in the emergency room or on an ambulance or rescue. The hands-on application of knowledge to real-life situations is critical, since books can teach basic concepts, but can't compare to the challenges of dealing with real patients in real emergency situations.

During my first semester of EMT school, I began my emergency room shifts at a small ER in downtown Orlando. I arrived an hour early, eager to get started. The physician on staff turned out to be an excellent teacher, letting me shadow him throughout the morning as he interviewed and treated patients. I took blood pressures, bandaged wounds, and assisted him with suturing. The morning flew by and before I knew it, it was early afternoon and I had yet to break for breakfast or lunch. I was walking out of the ER when the doctor called me into one of the examining rooms, saying he had an interesting case I might want to observe.

The patient, an elderly man lying face-down on the examining table, had come in with a large lump on his back between his shoulder blades. The doc explained to me it was a sebaceous cyst. Sebaceous cysts typically arise from swollen hair follicles. They form benign, enclosed sacs under the skin and are filled with an oily, foul-smelling, cheese-like substance. Of course, I didn't know all of this when I entered the room. I stood by as the nurse prepped the patient and the doctor assembled his equipment.

He began by injecting the cyst with a numbing agent. He applied this using a small syringe, making multiple injections into the lump. The injections caused small beads of blood to appear on the cyst, which the doc quickly wiped away using a piece of gauze. When the patient was thoroughly numb, he took a scalpel from the tray and made an incision across the cyst. It immediately began to ooze a mixture of blood and a yellowish substance that looked like cottage cheese. The first wave of nausea washed over me and I took a few deep breaths to try to clear my head.

The doc proceeded to squeeze the lump, forcing the cottage cheese out of the wound and onto the patient's back where it was quickly wiped away by the accommodating nurse. When I thought it couldn't get much worse, he then took a small pair of blunt-nosed scissors, stuck them directly into the incision, spread them open, and squeezed the remainder of the cheese from the lump. That was it. Suddenly, it was as if heavy, black curtains were closing in front of my eyes. My vision was reduced to a narrow hazy slit and my hearing was blotted out by the roar of rushing water in my ears. I knew the signs and symptoms of psychogenic shock, where a sudden draining of blood from the brain can induce unconsciousness. I knew I was about to experience it firsthand. I slowly backed out of the room, feeling my way down the short hallway and out into the small waiting room. The room was empty and I felt my way to a chair, tried putting my head between my knees, but was quickly overcome and passed out with my head against the wall, my legs splayed out in front of me.

I had fled to the waiting room with the hopes of remaining unobserved, noting the room was empty when I was leaving for lunch earlier. However, when I came to, I woke to a large panicked woman sitting next to me, screaming at the top of her lungs "She's having a seizure!! She's having a seizure!!"

Although I was confused, pale, and sweaty, I assured her I was all right, hoping to shut her up before she alerted the entire staff. Too late. The doctor, followed by two nurses and the receptionist, rushed into the waiting room, only to find me sitting there, pasty and humiliated. I explained what happened, and they assisted me to the restroom where I washed my face and collected myself. That was my introduction to the emergency room. That experience has served me well. As humiliating as it was, it taught me that when dealing with high-stress situations, control your breathing, keep your knees soft, and stay focused.

A BRAVE NEW WORLD

I DEVELOPED AN EARLY FASCINATION WITH TRAUMA. WHETHER IT was blunt force injuries from falls, penetrating injuries from shootings or stabbings, or dismemberments that accompany high-speed collisions, I was intrigued by injury patterns and the complex methods of treating someone with multisystem trauma. When it came time to begin riding in the field, I told my instructor I wanted as much action as possible, the busiest truck in the city. He advised me that if I wanted action, there was only one place to go: Orlando Fire Department's Rescue 2.

Station 2 was one of eleven fire stations that protected the city limits. The department was established in 1883 following a fire in a downtown dressmaker's shop. It began with six volunteers whose equipment consisted of a hose and reel, buckets to form a brigade, a painter's ladder, and a hand-drawn wagon with which to transport the equipment. Over its one hundred-plus year history, it has developed into one of the most progressive fire departments in the Southeast. Its emphasis on specialized training is reflected in the department's Special Teams, which include a Dive Team, a Hazardous Materials Team, a High Angle Rescue Team for elevated rescues, and a Heavy Rescue for specialized extrication scenarios. Rescue 2 was one of three units assigned to Station 2, located on Orlando's west side. The neighborhood, just blocks from historic downtown Orlando with its beautiful buildings and tourist attractions, is known for its violence and poverty. Shootings are a regular occurrence, and a large percentage of the emergency calls involve the sizable homeless population that wanders its streets.

I drove by the station the day before I was scheduled to ride. I wanted to check out the location, as well as see what an actual fire station looked like. So I cruised by like a stalker, casing the neighborhood. The station was surrounded by small businesses and shabby houses. People wandered the streets, many pushing their belongings in shopping carts or dragging them in large grocery bags. The station itself was a two-story white masonry building with an American flag out front and a homeless man asleep on the bench next to it. A tower truck was parked on the driveway in front of the station. It had its ladder extended high into the air as men worked around it, kneeling next to equipment as they completed their morning checkout.

The size and complexity of the rigs was intimidating and my belly tightened when I thought about reporting for my clinical. But I showed up the next day, Easter Sunday, timid and ignorant. Fortunately, the crews were friendly and unassuming, and they welcomed me inside with greetings and handshakes. They showed me around the equipment, explaining what each piece was used for and the various ways they were implemented to attack fires. The station consisted of a rescue, a fire engine ("engine") and a ladder truck (referred to at OFD as a "truck" or "tower"). Each person had an assigned position, and the tasks of each position depended on the type of incident. The interconnection of personnel and equipment fascinated me and I was instantly hooked.

OFD, like most departments in Florida, works a twenty-four-hour shift that begins at 8:00 A.M. and ends the same time the next morning. "Calls" are the emergencies and nonemergencies that the crews respond to. This term derives from two sources: an emergency incident typically enters the Dispatch Center in the form of a phone call and the Dispatch Center then "calls" out the station via emergency tones. A call is also referred to as a "run," the term being interchangeable. Each morning, crews exchange information as to the number of runs they had the previous shift. A busy shift as Station 2 can consist of up to twenty or more runs. The language of firefighting and EMS is full of jargon, acronyms, and slang, although it varies throughout the country.

Aside from my fascination with the trucks and equipment, I found the environment equally intriguing. The crews joked incessantly. They seemed to prey on each other's faults and weaknesses, and nothing was off limits. They teased each other about events of the previous shift, told stories about embarrassing episodes in the crew's past, and even made fun of each other's physical characteristics. From an anthropological point of view, it was like observing a foreign culture or secret society. There were unspoken rules of conduct, especially where rank was concerned, but it was an atmosphere of camaraderie and humor. That first day at Station 2 would direct the next twelve years of my life. That day was also the point at which my mother began to die.

LOSS

FOLLOWING MY GRADUATION FROM HIGH SCHOOL THREE YEARS PREviously, my mother had been diagnosed with breast cancer. It appeared not as a lump, but as a small indentation in her breast she happened to notice one morning in the mirror. She was diagnosed, had a radical mastectomy, and took chemotherapy for a year. It was a difficult year of illness, treatment, and hair loss. She pulled through that year with stoicism and grace, never revealing her fears and frustrations.

For three years she was fine. Her exams and scans were negative and we had begun to breathe a bit easier. But then the vomiting started. For several months, it became increasingly difficult for her to keep food down. At first she brushed it off as indigestion. The family practitioner she worked for diagnosed it as esophagitis. How he could have ignored her past history astounds me to this day, knowing what I now know about the tendency for breast cancer to spread throughout the body. She began to lose weight, eventually becoming weak and anemic. She was taken to the ER the day I reported to Station 2. I called my father that afternoon to check on her condition, but all they could determine was that she was bleeding internally. The source of the bleed was a mystery. Thus began the last year of her life.

The cancer was back, having spread to her stomach and bones. There was little they could do other than treat the symptoms and try to keep her comfortable. She endured additional rounds of chemotherapy in hopes of slowing the disease's progression. Her lungs repeatedly filled with fluid, requiring several trips to the hospital during which chest tubes were inserted into her fragile body to enable her to breathe. Many of the patient assessment skills I learned in school I perfected on her. I learned about the "tented" skin and sunken eyes of hypovolemia, where lack of fluid in the body causes the skin to shrivel and loose its elasticity. I learned the difference between rales and rhonchi, various breath sounds caused by fluid buildup in the lungs. I also learned what it was like to deal with terminal patients. I divided my time between studying and taking care of her. She would die at home one year later on Christmas Day, two months after I became a medic. She was the first person I ever pronounced dead.

PART-TIMER

FOLLOWING MY FIRST DAY AT STATION 2, I IMMEDIATELY BEGAN researching the qualifications for becoming a firefighter. Through my research, I found out that there were smaller departments within Orange County that relied on part-time staff to augment their full-time personnel. The part-timers were paid per call and sometimes sponsored through the fire academy. The City of Maitland was one such department.

Maitland Fire Department is a small, well-funded department that provides fire and emergency medical services to the predominantly upper-middle-class residents of the municipality. The department consists of a single fire station located in the heart of its small downtown and relies on mutual aid responses from nearby county stations. The station houses an engine and rescue truck, with additional trucks (a ladder and brush truck) that respond to special incidents. The additional trucks are typically manned by part-time staff. The part-time staff can put in unlimited hours at the station or can respond to the station from home when the full-time personnel are called out on emergencies.

I had been told that if I went to work for Maitland FD, they would pay my way through the fire academy and I would be able to get on-the-job training in the meantime. I immediately applied. The hiring process for part-time personnel was a scaled-down version of a formal process. Since many of the part-time applicants were EMTs but not certified firefighters, they were tested on basic medical skills such as patient assessment. Each applicant was also assessed on strength and agility. Although the noncertified part-time personnel were not allowed to fight fire, they were still expected to work around the equipment. Applicants had to show that they could handle heavy equipment, scale a ladder, and perform basic skills using firefighting equipment and tools. If the applicant passed both of these sections, he or she was granted an interview. I passed both of the initial tests easily and sat down for my interview in front of personnel representing each rank on the department—a firefighter, an engineer, a lieutenant, and the deputy chief of the department. At the end of the interview, when asked what my goal in the fire service was, I naively replied, "To work for Orlando Fire Department." Although surprised by my candor, I think they respected the fact that I wasn't going to bullshit my way through the interview. My mother instilled in me the importance of honesty and frankness. Thirteen years later, those values would play a role in the demise of my career.

TRAINING DAY

There comes a point in every new firefighter's career when he or she must face the first training fire. Mine came when Maitland was invited to participate in a "live fire training" with several surrounding county agencies.

The training fire was held at a large, three-story wooden hotel in the rural town of Zellwood. Here several agencies got together to spare the owner the expense of having his less-than-profitable hotel demolished. Instead, they would make it a learning experience for inexperienced grunts like myself by giving us a taste of real fire.

The day was hot and muggy and we assembled around the dilapidated structure, laying out our gear. Numerous fire trucks were parked in haphazard arrangement throughout the lot. The hotel sat amid open, yellow fields, with large oaks throwing mottled shade across the surrounding grounds. While we readied ourselves for entry, training personnel gathered wooden pallets and bundles of hay, stuffing them into the rooms of the hotel where they would soon be lit off. They would then send us in and watch as the building was consumed around us. It was our job to take from the experience what we could and apply it later to real-life situations. My hands were shaking.

I had been reading everything I could about fire tactics, practicing with my gear so that I could blend in with the veterans. They sauntered among the units, greeting each other with casual nods, occasionally turning their heads to spit into the high grass, a gesture of bravado among men. I stayed close to my unit, going over my equipment and checking the level of air in my tank for the tenth time.

They lit off the structure several times throughout the day, as "companies" took turns entering the building and attacking the fire. Some carried specialized tools and practiced the high-paced destruction of forcible entry. Other teams were assigned to search the building for "victims"—weighted dummies dressed in worn-out fire gear, simulating one of our own overcome by smoke. It was their job to get the dummy out into fresh air. After each evolution, the men would sit back and rest, evaluating and criticizing the teams that followed.

I was assigned to the nozzle. This meant I was responsible for entering with my crew, finding the "seat" of the fire, and attacking it before it found its way into the attic where it could race unseen above our heads. Our entry was on the third floor. We quickly climbed an outside stairwell composed of rusted, dilapidated metal, certain it would fail with each step as we made our way upward. The weight of the gear, compounded by the fear pounding within my chest, had me gasping by the time we reached the top. We crouched on the upper platform, outside the door that led into a long, narrow hallway. We raced to get our masks on, the rush of air from our tanks cool and invigorating. I took several deep breaths and tried to slow my bounding pulse.

We entered the long hallway. Through the smoke we could barely make out the arrangement of the small rooms, which fed off the main hallway on either side. We crawled forward and could see flames flashing in the distance. The search teams entered with us, simultaneously searching each room as we approached the seat of the fire. I tried to take in all that was happening around me: the intense heat as we inched down the hallway and the shouts of men as they coordinated their search. A surreal cloud enveloped us, giving the scene a dreamlike quality as if underwater.

We approached the end of the hallway, where the training instructors had gorged the room with combustibles. The fire had broken free, funneling into the hallway and dancing across the ceiling above our heads. I stared in amazement at the canopy of flames that rushed toward us, seemingly intent on encircling our huddled mass. At my lieutenant's signal, I opened the nozzle, releasing 150 gallons of water per minute onto the fire and watching with disappointment as it retreated and disappeared. The sensation was like crushing a rare butterfly, erasing its beauty for the sake of some inner desire to destroy it.

We chased the fire down the hall, showered by water and debris from the deteriorating walls, and finally making entry into one of the rooms near the end of the hall. In another wing of the building, another of the fires that had been lit burst from its confines, breaking into the attic, where it could have full run of the structure. In no time, it was out of control, as crews raced behind it in an attempt to squelch its progress. Before we knew it, the attic was fully involved, the fire roaring above our heads. We backed down the hallway to that crumbling stairway, our radios blaring with high-pitched orders to evacuate.

We inched our way back down the crumbling staircase, wrestling the charged line as we made our way to the ground. Once down, we stood back and watched, trying to catch our breath, trying to appear calm. The hotel grew torchlike, consuming one hundred years of Florida history.

CLASS #64

To become a firefighter in the state of Florida, a candidate must meet the qualifications set forth by the Bureau of Fire Standards and Training. When I entered the field, the Minimum Standards Class that trained and certified firefighters was just over two months in length. One could also opt for a part-time course, taught at night or on weekends. The Central Florida Fire Academy was located at the city's technical institute. A class would begin in the fall, but I was already registered to begin paramedic school. Through luck or fate, the paramedic course was postponed and I managed to slide into the single vacancy at the academy. Ironically, it had been vacated by another female who had been forced to drop out at the last minute due to illness. I gladly took her spot, becoming the only female among a class of twenty-seven males. We would make up Class #64. I took it as a good omen that the class number was the year of my birth. The class would be my introduction to the competitive world of firefighting, my first experience in a male-dominated profession.

Knowing I would be starting the academy, I utilized my clinicals at OFD to learn as much as I could about firefighting. The crews were helpful and willingly shared their wisdom and experience with me. I trained extensively, running several miles each day and lifting weights. I relished the physical and emotional challenges.

The first day of the academy was my first experience in a paramilitary organization, but it was not my first exposure to the rigid structures of rank. Growing up the daughter of a naval captain, my childhood had been dictated by the U.S. Navy. As my class assembled in the gymnasium, the instructors strolled in front of the group, surveying the lot. The instructors were seasoned veterans, qualified by experience and their ability to intimidate. They lined us up, looking us over with subtle scorn, deciding to themselves who would sink and who would swim. One of the older, "saltier" instructors strode to the center of the gym. He then made a statement that would fuel my determination for the remainder of the course.

In a booming, southern drawl he said, "We'll lose over a third of you. The two most obvious are the big guy and the girl." He eyeballed the overweight kid at the other end of the line before settling his intimidating gaze on me. I didn't move. I felt the eyes of the class on me, my stomach a coil of nerves and fear. But I met his gaze without blinking, thinking to myself "We'll see, asshole."

Teaching methods at the fire academy were different from any I had encountered at the university. For one thing, university professors don't make their students perform twenty push-ups for an incorrect response. It was initially humiliating to get up in front of the entire class and pump out push-ups, especially being the only female in the group. I was self-conscious of my body, the way I walked, and the fact that all eyes were on me when I went to the front of the room. But I overcame those feelings, masking them with self-confidence. I learned to adapt, taking my lumps like everyone else.

Each day would begin with an hour of physical training (PT). We would assemble in the gymnasium and the instructors would bark orders as our class of sweating grunts pumped out push-ups, sit-ups, and a variety of calisthenics. The instructors would wander among our ranks, criticizing our form, blowing their whistles in our ears when we weren't performing up to snuff, making fun of each of us as clueless rookies who had obviously chosen the wrong profession. They constantly reminded us why we shouldn't be there. Some of us were too slow. Others lacked coordination. I was singled out for "being a girl." On the rare occasion my performance was praised, it was always tagged with the phrase ". . . for a girl." But each of us took the verbal abuse in stride, and over time, the instructors became less intimidating, many of them taking on the role of mentor.

Once we completed our indoor exercises, we would head outside to run laps around the training field. The run was usually accompanied by a series of groans emanating from the ranks. The instructors would chase us like dogs, barking out orders to "Speed up!" "Get your heads out of your asses!" and my favorite, "Come on you bunch of pansies!" We approached the runs with a combination of dread and humor. We knew it was something we would have to endure each morning for the next two months. Whining about it was pointless.

The academy curriculum was designed to transform a student from complete ignorance to moderate competency in fighting fires and handling emergency scenes. We learned how to handle the multitude of tools used in forcible entry, vehicle extrication, and fire suppression. We drilled continuously, running stairs with heavy packs on our shoulders and collapsing in exhaustion when we reached the ground. We dragged each other around to simulate patient removal from hazardous situations, and we learned to control hoses from which hundreds of gallons per minute flowed. Like any field in which timing is critical, our training focused on repetition and "muscle memory." Tasks were to become automatic so that on a fire scene, when seconds count, the body reacts and functions in a controlled, expedient manner. This minimizes errors on the fire ground and ensures smooth operations as emergency situations unfold.

The class learned quickly, and within several weeks, we were able to function as a semicoherent group while drilling on the training ground. On those frequent occasions when we lost our concentration or stumbled over one another while trying to complete a task, the instructors would shout at us in tones reserved for incompetents.

"You worthless sons of bitches! Give me five laps!"

Whatever task we were mangling would come to a screeching halt as we slowly made our way to the field to run laps in full gear. We looked like parading clowns, running around the training field in boots, coats, and helmets, although it made our morning runs seem like easy jaunts in comparison.

Among anthropologists who study rites of passage, the "liminal" period is a time when individuals are transitioning between two different states. They have lost their original identity, but have yet to achieve their new status. It is a state of "in between." Those transitioning together between identities form a "communitas," a social structure based on equality where bonds form, tying the individuals together as they progress through the process. I saw this firsthand at the academy. We became a fairly tight-knit group during our weeks of training, bound to each other in an effort to make it through successfully.

Although I felt a part of the group, there was always that degree of separation imposed by gender. Each time I split from the group to go to my locker room, hearing the laughter and conversations of the men as they went to theirs, I felt left out of the closeness they shared, the familiarity among them. Although they accepted me as a fellow student, I would never be a true member of the "brotherhood." I accepted this with resignation, feeling I could at least gain acceptance through hard work and determination. I felt if they saw I was serious, that I was intent on being the best I could be, that any reservations they had concerning my abilities would dissipate and I would be considered one of them. I tried to adhere to these beliefs throughout my career. As optimistic as I was, the "brotherhood" would remain an impenetrable boundary.

By graduation, our class had shrunk by a third. We lost a few following our live fire training, which took place in a small "burn building" in a neighboring county. The building was constructed to resemble a two-story residence, but was made of flame-resistant materials that could tolerate the intense heat of training fires. The structure was rudimentary compared to the high-tech burn buildings of today

The day of our live burn, the class was loaded into a dilapidated school bus for the two-hour ride into the country. The day was clear and we were nervous. Many of us had never experienced live fire before. I had participated in the joint training operation with Maitland, so I was a bit more prepared, but all of us were tense, joking loudly to hide our anxiety.

When we arrived at the structure, we spread our gear in the high grass that surrounded the building, lining up each piece in the order in which it would be "donned." The instructors prepared the building, loading the pallets that would be lit off as our teams made entry.

The live burn served as the culmination of our training. As the evolutions unfolded, we applied the skills we had learned during our training to the tasks of combating the fire. One of the skills we applied that day was dealing with situations involving tight spaces. What prepared us was the maze.

The "smoke maze" is a confusing series of tunnels you crawl through on hands and knees, sometimes sliding sideways in order to squeeze your oversized, encumbered frame through the narrow opening of each segment. In this timed drill, you enter the maze blindfolded and in full gear, breathing from your tank, your helmet strapped tightly to your head. It's like trying to crawl through a narrow tunnel while wrapped in a heavy quilt. There are wires and ropes strung throughout the maze that are designed to ensnare the tank on your back or wrench the helmet from your head. The tunnels are constructed so that the floor of the maze changes elevation constantly. At times you find yourself crawling up steps, then having to cautiously lower yourself until the floor resumes beneath you. This emphasizes the importance of "sweeping" the floor before you to prevent falling through a burned-out hole.

Then there are the hidden pockets where instructors crouch in the darkness, waiting for the opportunity to reach through openings in the maze to turn off your air supply. You're crawling along in the dark, panting, your heart racing, when suddenly you go to breathe: *No air!* This usually takes place in the tightest confines of the maze, when you're unable reach behind you to turn your tank back on. You are forced to backtrack, frantically forcing your body backwards until you come to a spot wide enough to allow the reach. By then, you're panicked from lack of air, your mask sucked tight against your face as you strain for the slightest breath.

The maze is designed to force a firefighter to deal with the anxiety that accompanies being wedged into extremely tight spots. Some don't make it. They are overcome by claustrophobia and begin to panic, their gear becoming increasingly constricting the more they struggle. Claustrophobia usually breaks a few candidates in each class. They just can't keep themselves calm and it spells the end of their dreams of fighting fire.

When it comes to actual firefighting, the ability to "talk yourself down" and avoid panic is essential. The more frustrated you become the greater the panic, a situation that quickly spirals downward. Many firefighters have died after becoming trapped or lost, panicking when they realize they have a limited supply of air and can't remember their way out or become entangled within a structure. I remember reading about a firefighter killed in a house fire after his air tank became entangled in a bicycle. Anything can catch you up.

So we train extensively in preparation for the real thing. We lost two candidates the day of the live burn, one of them the overweight kid that had been singled out with me at the beginning of the class. The other decided he just wasn't cut out for the job.

At graduation, we stood proudly as our certificates were presented. Various awards were handed out: best performance on the training ground, highest grade point average. I had broken the sit-ups record at the academy, beating it by performing one hundred sit-ups in 90 seconds. My name was engraved on a plaque that hung in the hallway of the academy. I would visit it from time to time over the next few years when attending special training courses, proud to see my name on the wall. It was eventually broken many years later by an annoying triathlete.

Following graduation from the academy, I returned to the community college to begin my first semester of paramedic school. It was a relief to be in a college classroom again. I excelled in my coursework and devoured the curriculum, carrying my books with me everywhere. I was anxious to return to the emergency room as a paramedic student where I would be let loose to practice the advanced techniques I was learning in class. As paramedic students, we were allowed to move from the smaller, quieter ERs into the action-packed environment of the trauma center. My first night there would stick with me for the rest of my career.

THE TRAUMA ROOM

Orlando Regional Medical Center is one of seven Level I trauma centers in the state of Florida and is located just south of downtown. According to the 2007 Alliance to Save Florida's Trauma Centers, a Level I trauma center is a "State-designated center capable of delivering the highest level of expertise and care in the shortest possible time, with capabilities that far exceed a non-trauma center hospital." They provide a range of specialists, such as neuro, thoracic, and orthopedic surgeons available around the clock and have special facilities for treating burns and pediatrics.

When it comes to treating traumatic injuries, emergency personnel operate under the rule of the "Golden Hour," which begins at the time of the injury and ends when the patient receives definitive care, preferably at a trauma center. It is the responsibility of EMS personnel to stabilize and treat patients and then transport them expediently to the closest appropriate hospital, preferably a Level I facility. In trauma, every minute counts.

My first night as a paramedic student in the trauma center was not a pleasant experience. I chose a Friday, one of their busiest nights. Business typically booms as people go out drinking and driving, doing the drugs they have been saving for all week, or carrying out earlier threats of violence.

I arrived early in the evening and the ER was already full. Patients were stretched out on beds in the hallway and the waiting area was filled to capacity.

Emergency rooms treat all sorts of people. That's what makes the work so interesting. But an emergency room located in one of the prime tourist areas in the United States offers an even greater variety of race, religion, and socio-economic status. Although variety is abundant, the poor still make up the majority of patients. The ER is their only source of medical care aside from the overcrowded free clinics that are usually closed on the weekends.

I spent my first hour trying to stay out of the nurses' way as they flew between beds, trying to appease the patients that had been waiting for hours for test results, prescriptions, or to speak to a doctor. The majority of the physicians were young residents, many fresh out of medical school. The trauma center also served as a teaching hospital, providing a training ground for inexperienced interns. They learned quickly.

I tried to make myself useful, but the nurses seemed too overwhelmed to take a moment to allow me to attempt any of my required skills. These included drawing blood, starting intravenous lines, and assessing patients. One of the older nurses finally took pity on me, instructing me in short sentences to grab my equipment and follow her.

I was to draw blood and start an IV on a patient whose apprehension increased when he noticed the fear in my eyes and the subtle shaking of my hands. As I set up my equipment, I asked the nurse if I should use an 18-gauge needle to draw the blood. She replied sarcastically "Would you appreciate an 18 gauge needle in your arm?" By the curt tone of her voice, I guessed I wouldn't, but I had already opened the needle and didn't want to appear even more uncertain. So I proceeded with the IV and blood draw and fortunately met with success. I left the patient's side and quietly blended in with the chaos of the unit.

The night continued at its hectic pace and I became more assertive with each hour, practicing on unsuspecting patients and making small checks on my skills list. Just as the workload was easing, a trauma alert was called for an infant in cardiac arrest. This would turn out to be one of the most violent cases of my career.

The doors to the unit flew open as EMS personnel raced in, leaning over a small figure on their stretcher as they performed chest compressions in an attempt to circulate blood through its small body. I had never seen CPR performed on an infant and the mechanics of it amazed me as the medics aggressively, yet gently, continued resuscitation.

They entered the trauma room, the primary room designated for the worst cases. It contained all the necessary equipment to treat a traumatically injured patient, from prepackaged surgical kits to sterilized tools used to crack chests. They transferred the small patient onto the bed as the team of doctors and nurses began barking orders to each other in an attempt to restart the baby's heart.

The baby had not been sick. It had no preexisting conditions. It was in the trauma center because its father had been fighting with its mother and knew the best way to hurt her would be to hurt the infant. He had forced her from the baby's room, locked the door, and gone to work. She frantically ran from the house, screaming for help from neighbors and running to the window of the infant's room. She arrived in time to see the father pick the infant up by the ankles and swing it against the bedroom wall.

The baby never had a chance. It sustained massive head injuries that quickly stopped the heart, injuries that now turned it a mottled blue. Its deadened gaze peered out from its swollen head as the ER staff tried in vain to save it.

It was hard to take in. The chaos of the scene, the description of the events, and the extent of the baby's injuries were overwhelming. After an hour of resuscitative efforts, I fled from the room. I found a dark corner in the hospital where I fought back tears, humiliated at my weakness. They eventually restarted the heart but by this time, the brain had been without oxygen for so long that the electroencephalograph administered the following morning showed flat brain waves, and life support was discontinued.

I thought about that infant for days, trying to force it from my mind, yet reliving the incident in order to learn what I could from the resuscitative measures. I was in awe of the concerted efforts of the emergency room staff and the speed at which tasks were performed. But I was horrified at the level of violence inflicted on the small child. I knew I had chosen a career in which such scenes were the norm. I wasn't disheartened. I knew with each incident I would become more immune to the suffering, more immune to the trauma, and more accepting of the atrocities that humans inflict on one another.

HOSPITAL ROTATIONS

The months wore on and I completed my first semester of paramedic school. During this time, my mother's health deteriorated. My progress through school was paralleled by her declining health, as if they were two converging paths: my increase in medical knowledge and the wasting of her slight frame. The more I learned, the more I came to recognize her impending death. In the emergency room and in the field, I was confronted by other terminal patients. I recognized the same exhaustion in their eyes, the look of quiet resignation that eventually sets in.

The months of school are a blur to me now. When I think back to that period, it's as if time existed in shadows, where only a hint of memory plays across my mind. What I do remember are my hospital rotations.

Paramedic students, like medical school interns, are required to complete a number of hours in various departments within the hospital. These include the emergency room, of course, but also pediatrics, respiratory therapy, the burn unit (which was horrifying), and obstetrics (OB). The OB ward was one of the most entertaining of my rotations.

I spent the day rushing behind frantic interns as they delivered squealing infants into the hands of exhausted new mothers. But the most dramatic moment was watching an emergency Cesarean section.

The woman was rushed into the delivery room, flanked by the OB staff and accompanied by a neonate team, since the baby wasn't due for another month. The woman was suffering from eclampsia, a dangerous condition involving high blood pressure and seizures. Treatment for the condition is immediate delivery of the baby. The team was wasting no time. The woman's swollen abdomen was quickly prepped, a large brown swath of Betadine smeared across her extended belly. The lead physician took scalpel in hand as I stood by at the foot of the bed, anxiously awaiting the large incision he would make from one side of her lower abdomen to the other.

He cut through the outer layers of skin, exposing the mass of muscle overlying the uterus. He carefully but swiftly cut through the layers of muscle before finally penetrating the uterus. As he cut into the uterus, a spray of amniotic fluid flew out of the mother, sailing right past my head as I dodged to avoid being hit. He reached into her belly, pulling from it a shriveled form and immediately handing it off to the awaiting neonate team. In a moment, the baby was squealing, the mother was smiling, and everyone was taking a deep breath.

It was one of the most astounding procedures I've ever seen. It made normal deliveries seem simplistic. In a normal delivery, the mother does all the work and all we have to do is deliver the newborn without dropping it. That day stands out in my mind as a unique experience in the life of a student, one that would prepare me for the four babies I would eventually deliver in the field as a medic.

Of all the rotations, the worst for me was respiratory therapy (RT). If you ask medical personnel what bothers them the most about working with sick people, they can quickly fire off their least favorite thing, such as shit, vomit, or blood. Mine is mucus. For some reason, I've always loathed phlegm. I can stand any amount of blood, I can even tolerate someone vomiting on my shoes, but if I'm up against a big wad of snot, I'm a goner. I found this out while spending time shadowing a respiratory therapist during my clinical rotations.

I arrived in the RT department, skills sheet in hand. I was to complete some of the more rudimentary skills of airway control, primarily handling various airway devices and suctioning. I would perform intubations later under the guidance of an anesthetist in the operating room. On that day, my main goal was to suction an intubated patient using sterile technique, since this is rarely done in the field.

The respiratory therapist (also referred to as an RT) ushered me into the room of a comatose patient who was being ventilated via a stoma. A stoma is a small round opening that is placed in the neck of the patient and provides direct access into the trachea. Therefore, breathing bypasses the upper airway. A permanent airway device, they are frequently used on comatose patients and allow more direct access to the respiratory tract. The problem is they become clogged with mucus and must be suctioned frequently, depending on the condition of the patient. This patient was waging a serious battle with phlegm.

The direct access to the respiratory tract requires suctioning be performed using sterile technique. I assembled my equipment at the bedside, donning sterile gloves and carefully handling the skinny, flexible plastic tubing that I would advance into the stoma and down into his trachea. I prepped the stoma by wiping it with an alcohol prep, feeling a tightening in my stomach as I began suctioning the gooey, opaque mucus from the stoma's opening. I then advanced the tubing down into his trachea, as the suction unit began its nauseating slurp. Placing my finger over the opening in the side of the tubing that allows suction to build in the tube, I twisted the tubing between my fingers as I pulled it up and out of the airway so that it would suction the sides of the trachea on its way out. Holding my breath and counting the seconds until it was over, I was just finishing the procedure when, to my horror, I pulled out the end of the tube on which a large greenish hunk of phlegm hung quivering. I panicked, removing my finger from the opening in the tube, which immediately released suction. The large blob fell from the end of the tubing and landed on the patient's chest with a wet "Slap!"

That was it! I gagged loudly, trying to hold onto my breakfast as my throat convulsed. I managed to keep everything down as the RT looked on with mild amusement. From that day on, mucus would become my sworn enemy. It would come back to haunt me a year later when treating a patient who had suffered double strokes.

The patient was at home recovering from a previous stroke when she was struck with a second. The initial stroke had left her unable to move her right side. The second stroke knocked out movement on the left. She was completely helpless, unable to move any of her extremities.

We loaded her into the ambulance and I placed her on oxygen and attached the cardiac monitor. She was stable and talkative, so after starting an IV, I sat back to jot a few notes on my report. That was when she started clearing her throat. It wasn't a delicate throat clearing. It was one of those efforts that originate deep in the chest, accompanied by a noisy upwelling of snot. I asked her if she was all right and she said she needed to spit. I placed a small pile of 4x4 bandages in my hand and held it to her mouth. She then hawked a large goober the size of an oyster into my hand as the familiar sensation of the dry heaves erupted in my belly. She continued noisily clearing her airway as I held the 4x4s to her face, the whole time leaning behind the head of the stretcher, retching violently. By the time we arrived at the hospital, my stomach was a coiled knot, my partner in stitches from laughing the entire way.

A RAINY SUNDAY

Before I knew it, my coursework was complete and I was preparing for the state exam. I passed with a 97 and was released to my "provisional" period, where I would ride with other licensed medics and work toward completing another advanced list of skills. These included performing airway intubations, defibrillating patients in cardiac arrest, starting IVs, and administering medications.

It was one of those rainy Sunday mornings; red lights flashed over empty streets and animals kept to their dry places. I had spent the morning over steaming cups of coffee, combing the paper for relevant news and refreshing my memory on the anatomy of the airway and the proper dosage of Valium for a seizing child.

The call came later, to one of the elite neighborhoods tucked among giant oaks and brick-lined streets. The home was set back from the road, a large two-story house bathed in the subtle colors of the wealthy. We were called to a shooting, but it was out of place: the wrong neighborhood, wrong time of day, wrong day of the week. Who shoots somebody on a Sunday morning? Usually shootings come late on those hot, violent summer nights when people are bored and angry, looking for a release from all those years of eating cheap, processed food and taking the bus instead of driving. This call was wrong from the beginning.

We entered the house amid chaos. The police were milling around, looking busy and uncomfortable as the parents wailed in grief, pounding the arms of the officers for answers as to why they came home and found their young son lying face up in their walk-in closet with their revolver in his hand and his brains in a grainy, red stain on the wall.

We climbed the stairs, merging with the firefighters who were already there. I eased my way past their large frames and into the closet full of fine clothes and designer shoes. He was stretched out on the floor, a boy of about twelve. He was dressed in a pair of swim trunks, as if he had spent the morning deciding whether to brave the harsh weather for a swim or dig through his parents' closet for the gun they kept hidden. He had obviously chosen the latter, for there he was, his dead eyes staring up at the ceiling as we rushed around, trying to ventilate him, trying to establish intravenous lines, trying to keep what was left of his head from spilling out onto the shoes lined up neatly next to him.

I prodded long-collapsed veins on his small, pale arms, wondering to myself what had brought him to this point on a rainy Sunday morning, the point where nothing else matters but escape. Not the bewilderment of friends, the pain and failure of parents, just the release into the black unknown. Away from the dark fears that wake you in the early hours of the morning and creep around the bedside, gently pulling on the covers so that they move just enough to feel it against your skin.

We never established the intravenous lines, but managed to contain what remained of his head, wrapping it in bulky, white dressings, the kind of bandaging you see on ridiculous dramas where the person wakes up clear-headed after years of coma. We lifted his slight frame onto the stretcher, carrying it down the stairs and through the beautiful house. His parents stared on in horror, wondering where they had gone wrong, furious at him for putting them in such a socially compromising position, wondering how they would ever explain this at the club and whether their friends would ever believe them when they said they had no idea he was in pain.

We transported him to the hospital, the lights from our truck cutting through steady rain. As we entered the trauma room, the staff of young surgeons looked on. The reality of the situation was written on their faces, deeply lined from the sleepless night they had spent trying to save the victims of last night's violence. As we placed the boy on the table, they descended like a team huddling up before a play. The least tired of them took the lead, calling out orders to the nurses who flew among the room like moths, grabbing trays of surgical tools, cutting the faded trunks from the boy's body, exposing his fragile genitalia.

They knew immediately it was hopeless. The boy had been without a pulse for over thirty minutes, and what had previously been his brain was either splashed on the closet wall or seeping into the bulky bandages encircling his head. They looked at each other, exchanging information without saying a word, until one of them finally announced the time of death.

We filtered out of the room, my partners and I to attend to the mess in the back of the ambulance, the surgeons on to better, salvageable patients. I did what I do after every gruesome call. I flashed through the events, critiquing my own actions and those around me, forming a mental list of the things I would have done differently and the things I would repeat. I pushed from my mind his young, blank eyes, the slightness of his frame that would never grow to adulthood, those small hands that had pulled on that faded pair of trunks then pulled a gun from the closet. I busied myself with the tasks at hand, filing him away with all the other nameless deaths that floated within my subconscious.

The day should have ended there. We should have had a quiet afternoon in which we would return to the subject of the boy from time to time, commenting on the shock of the parents, the mess of the closet, discussing plans for dinner. But the afternoon turned busy and soon we were scrambling through the city answering the calls of the desperate and the bored.

We arrived on the scene of an elderly woman complaining of chest pain. She was distraught, as many of our elderly patients are. We typically dote on them for a while, trying to make them comfortable, easing their fears and touching them gently. But there was something different about this call. Her family stood by looking worried and scared, several of the younger ones cowering in the hallway with tears on their faces, looking at us with quiet desperation.

It was puzzling. Cardiac calls were regular events and usually it took oxygen and a nitro tablet to calm the patient and ease their chest pain. But this woman was truly distraught, the kind of anguish nothing we carried could ease. So as my partner tried to calm her, I searched the room for evidence of who she was, what her life was like from day to day, looking for medicine bottles, food containers, surveying the overall cleanliness of the place.

As my eyes combed the room, I couldn't help noticing the family members again. They were acting as if she had already died. As if they had found her this morning, cold and stiff in bed. Something wasn't right. So I continued my investigation when something on her bookshelf caught my eye. I scanned the faded pictures of her when she was young and had future plans. Among the shelves were colorful photos of grandchildren in their finest clothes but resembling most school pictures—hair and clothes in disarray because the children were called in from recess to sit down, sweaty and anxious, and have their picture taken so their parents could distribute them to lonely relatives. One picture stuck out among the others. It was a beautiful young boy sitting up straight in a crisp, white shirt and an oversized tie, smiling into the camera. He had a particular depth to his eyes and something about him was strangely familiar.

In an instant, the events of the day came rushing toward me with such force I could hear the roar of it in my ears. The previous call flashed through my brain with violent rapidity, leaving me stunned and silent. I was looking into the smiling face of the boy I had worked on earlier that day, the one who had lay down in his parents' closet, held the gun to his head, and pulled the trigger, never saying good-bye to the people who now had come to give the news to the grandmother that her beautiful grandchild just couldn't cope and had escaped from all his fears that morning.

THE TEST

My goal from the start had been to work for OFD. As an EMT student new to the field of EMS, I listened closely to conversations of firefighters from various departments. I quickly perceived that OFD was one of the top departments in the state, with an extensive history, great benefits, and vicious competition for each position. Hiring cycles for OFD took place approximately every two years, based on demand and retirements within the department. Each of these "cycles" would consist of hundreds of applicants vying for a limited number of positions. I knew I was in for some stiff competition.

I had trained extensively to prepare myself for the academy. My training increased significantly in preparation for OFD's hiring process. I ran almost every day, spent almost each morning in the gym when I wasn't in class, and knew I would have to be in the best shape possible to achieve a high score on the skills portion of the process.

Most competitive fire departments have hiring processes that consist of three phases: a written test to gauge the candidate's knowledge of basic firefighting practices and tactics, a physical agility test to gauge fitness, and a "skills" portion that consists of various fire-ground operations. This includes air pack drills, laddering buildings, advancing hose lines, search and rescue, and any number of tasks that test a candidate's knowledge and agility on a fire scene. OFD's skills test was notorious for weeding out the weak and rewarding only those with the determination and drive of pit bulls.

The hiring process was separated into phases. It began with a written exam and physical agility test, which were completed on the same day. Applicants who passed both sections would return a week later to participate in the skills portion of the process. I scored a 98 on written exam, having studied my Fire Standards text until I had large chunks of it memorized. The physical agility test required the applicant to perform the same exercises performed at the fire academy: namely push-ups, sit-ups, running, grip strength, and measurement of body fat. I did well on the test, maxing out on push-ups and sit-ups and gleefully moving on to the next stage, the skills assessment.

I had heard horror stories about OFD's skills assessment test. It was notorious for being one of the most difficult assessments in the state, and I had gotten wind that they were trying out a new test that pushed the candidates even harder than previous assessments. These assessments are especially challenging for females, who typically lack the body mass and upper-body strength required to complete the tasks within the required time limits. At the time, OFD had only six females in a department of over 350, an incredibly small number compared to departments of similar size. That was due in large measure to the difficulty of their skills assessment tests.

The skills assessment was set up in "stations" where a candidate was tested on various aspects of the job. The applicant had to move through each phase of the assessment without stopping. This ensured physical exhaustion of the candidates, a rudimentary form of natural selection. The stations began benignly enough. Assessment of medical skills and ropes and knots progressed on to the more physically demanding stages of the test. The air pack drill required the candidate to assemble and don protective gear in under two minutes. The third station, the ladder exercise, consisted of "throwing" a twenty-four-foot ladder against a building and advancing it into a second story window, gathering tools and a hose line, and getting yourself and the equipment up and into the window, all the while using proper technique. The candidate was dressed in full gear and air pack, which saddled you with an extra eighty pounds, not including the tools and hose line.

Next was the "smoke maze." Any tendencies toward claustrophobia usually surface when performing the maze. Thus, it is used as another weeding-out mechanism at most assessments. I, however, had always enjoyed the challenges of the maze and became proficient during the fire academy. I completed OFD's maze in record time, the fastest of any of the female candidates.

But I was battling an additional challenge that day. I had originally been scheduled to complete the skills assessment the previous week. However, I had come down with a stomach virus and for three days had been sidelined with vomiting and diarrhea. The illness had left me weak and shaky. I had dropped five pounds, but felt confident that if I choked down a carbohydrate-laden plate of pasta and eggs the morning of the assessment, I could push through the test. However, the effects of the illness would catch up with me during the search-and-rescue portion of the exam.

Following the maze, the candidate was immediately escorted to a darkened room where two 150-pound sand-filled dummies were hidden among overturned furniture and debris. Still blindfolded and panting from the maze, the candidate enters the room, performs a right-hand search, locating each dummy and dragging it out to the safety of the hallway. The exercise ends when the applicant "tags" the door: hanging a search tag on the door handle to indicate the room is clear of victims.

I knew I was in trouble during the ladder exercise. By the time I got to the top, my legs were weak and shaking. At 5'7" and 135 pounds (following my virus-induced weight loss plan), I was strong but lacked the bulk to power my way through the test. After completing the maze, my adrenaline stores were depleted and I could feel my strength fading rapidly. I entered the search floor and my time started.

I located the first of the dummies, which were large human-shaped beanbags with nothing to grab hold of. I ended up putting the dummy in a headlock and pulling with all I had. This would not have been proper technique in real life, but for the purpose of the exam, a candidate was allowed to use any means possible to get the dummies out the door. I got the first one through the door and rested for a moment on all fours, trying desperately to catch my breath. I didn't think I had the strength to enter the room a second time.

Fortunately, one of my academy instructors, a lieutenant with OFD, was overseeing that phase of the assessment. He knew I was determined to work for OFD, so he screamed in my ear "Either get off your ass or go home!" I realized this was it. This was my only opportunity to complete the test that I had trained months for, so I somehow dragged myself up from the floor by grasping the door handle and made my way back into the dark room.

I don't remember finding the second dummy. That portion of the test is blank in my mind. All I remember is arriving outside the door again, dropping the dummy at my feet, and trying to stay conscious. I still needed to tag the door, but I couldn't seem to make my arms work. Suddenly, a hand was grasping my wrist, guiding my hand up to my chest pocket where the door tags were held. That was enough to remind me to lift one of the tags from my pocket and hook it to the doorknob. I slapped it on the knob and the search was complete.

The instructors then led me to the stairwell to exit the training tower and move on to the final phase of the assessment. They checked my responsiveness by asking me simple questions. But exhaustion was consuming me and I found I couldn't verbalize my responses. Instead, I kept pointing in the direction of the exit, indicating I just wanted to finish the test. Luckily they complied and led me to the final stage.

The final station was a hose pull. The candidate had to drag a fully charged 150-foot section of hose about fifty feet, open the nozzle, strike two targets (which were basketballs placed on top of traffic cones), drag it another fifty feet, then hit a final target without collapsing in cardiac arrest.

A gallon of water weighs just over eight pounds. So the weight of a fifty-foot section of hose can be challenging to maneuver, especially when your arms and legs are shaking from exhaustion. I leaned into the hose line to try to get my weight behind it and it was like pushing a brick wall. I brought it over the back of my shoulder, laying it diagonally across my chest with the nozzle tucked under my left arm and pulled with everything I had. I managed to make it to the first cone, took aim, and somehow knocked the ball from its cone. I pivoted my position, opened the nozzle, and knocked the second ball from its perch. I then proceeded to the final target, my knees almost buckling each time I lunged forward. I centered myself, swung the nozzle up into position, and found I couldn't pull it open. My arms burned, my throat was parched, and every muscle fiber in my body was on fire. But somehow I managed, using repeated small hits against the lever of the nozzle, to open it and aim. The stream wavered, missing the ball initially, but with one last push I steadied the nozzle, knocking the ball from the cone.

The next thing I knew, multiple hands were on me, pulling my gear from my body and guiding me to a folding metal chair where I had my blood pressure and pulse checked. Like all the candidates, mine was through the roof, but I managed to pass and the exhilaration I felt walking away from that test was immeasurable.

TRAIN WRECK

TRAINS CAN BE DEVASTATING MACHINES, ESPECIALLY WHEN THEY GO up against the haphazard driving of an elderly man who thinks he and his aged Impala can beat the crossing gates. He and his car ended up several hundred feet from where he was struck, both destroyed by the impact. The train always wins.

I was still a provisional medic, riding the ambulance under the supervision of a seasoned paramedic while I completed my checklist of skills. Some of these skills can be difficult to obtain. You can go a long time without having the opportunity to perform some of the more advanced procedures. I was about to get a few of those skills checked off.

We arrived on the scene, which was located about one hundred yards down the track from the point of impact. We dragged our equipment and stretcher down the track to the wreck. The crushed remains of an older-model car sat sideways across the tracks, the overheated brakes of the train steaming nearby. The wreck occurred in the city of Maitland, where I had been working as a part-time firefighter. I knew the fire department personnel, who were struggling to free the patient's feet, which had become wedged up under the gas and brake pedals. There was extensive damage to the vehicle as well as the patient. The driver had ended up head-down, hanging out of the driver's side of the vehicle, his feet jammed up under the dash. Since intubation was a skill that can be hard to come by, I jumped at the opportunity, positioning myself next to what remained of the patient's face and setting up my equipment.

The man had extensive facial and head trauma. One of the paramedics continued to ventilate him as I readied my equipment. I then instructed him to back up so that I could position myself at the top of the patient's head. I inserted the blade of the laryngoscope into his mouth. A laryngoscope is a device used to open the airway, elevating the tongue and chin in order to visualize the vocal cords. However, proper placement of a laryngoscope depends on an intact chin, which on this patient had been crushed upon impact. In fact, his entire face had taken on a mushy consistency and each time I tried to visualize the cords, his mouth would quickly fill with blood from his extensive injuries. One of the medics suctioned his airway as I continued to ventilate him manually. The crushing injuries to his face were causing his frontal sinuses above the eyes to fill with blood. His condition was compounded by his inverted position. Each time I forced air into his lungs, a ribbon of blood would spray from the large gash in his forehead. It felt hopeless. He had been without a pulse for some time and his feet were still entrapped.

After several attempts, I advised the lieutenant that we needed to get orders from the hospital to stop resuscitation, since we were having no success establishing an airway. Protocols at that time gave rescuers the ability to obtain physician orders to stop resuscitative efforts when the patient met certain criteria deemed incompatible to life. The officer concurred and radioed the hospital to obtain the necessary orders. In the meantime, the firefighters continued their frantic rescue efforts. I fought with the mangled face while others took turns doing chest compressions. Another group struggled with the heavy equipment of extrication, trying to free the patient's feet from the crushed vehicle.

Word finally came over the radio allowing us to abandon our efforts, and I gratefully put down my equipment just as one of the lieutenants exclaimed that the feet were finally free. I gave him the signal that the resuscitation had been stopped, sliding a flattened hand across my throat, and I'll never forget the look of frustration and disappointment as he realized their efforts were in vain. We backed away from the patient, collecting our gear and beginning the slow task of cleaning up from the call.

Several days later, I attended my first Critical Incident Stress Debriefing, a technique used in the field to help personnel deal with traumatic calls so they don't end up babbling incoherently from stress years later. It was an intense session, as we sat in a large circle and took turns talking. We each explained our actions on the scene and the way we felt about the call in hindsight. As we proceeded around the circle, one of the dispatchers manning the radio at the time of the call began to speak. She had been on the job for many years, so I expected experience and professionalism. I was sadly disappointed. She proceeded to describe how frantic the Dispatch Center had been that day, all the phones ringing at once, and how stressed she still felt from having to juggle so many phone lines. I flashed back to the scene, remembering the frustration on the faces of the firefighters, the patient's blood striking my arms and chest, and the patient's crushed face as I attempted to oxygenate him. I would have taken a ringing phone over that any day.

LIFE ON AN AMBULANCE

WITH OFD'S HIRING PROCESS BEHIND ME, MY NAME WAS PUT ON A ranked list of candidates, and I awaited hire. I had completed my provisional phase as a medic and now worked for the private ambulance service in Orange County, honing my skills and biding my time. It was an excellent training ground. The call loads were heavy, since there were far fewer ambulances covering the county than there were fire stations. It was an exceptional learning experience, which lasted for about a year until I was hired by OFD.

I was assigned to a station located in a small hospital on Orlando's east side. Our quarters consisted of a hospital room equipped in the traditional manner with two single beds, a mounted television, and a small bathroom. My partner, George, was a quick-witted veteran who had worked in the field as an EMT for many years. He was well versed in EMS and could find humor in just about any situation. It made for easy shifts, even when we spent the majority of it in our truck.

Our territory stretched from the east side of downtown all the way to the St. Johns River, which serves as the county line. Some of our responses could stretch to twenty minutes or more, even with lights and sirens. During the day, we would chat and joke on our way to calls. I would sit with the map book in my lap to guide him into the scene, since computers and GPS hadn't arrived in EMS yet. He would sit beside me peering mischievously from behind the wheel as he expertly wove through traffic.

We had a great routine worked out for late-night calls. When we responded to the edge of the county, we had an understanding that I could sleep while he drove. Many times, I would feel a gentle nudge on my shoulder as he would wake me with "We're two minutes out." At that point, I would rub my eyes, trying to remember where we were going and the nature of the call.

It was early in the morning following a quiet night. We stumbled to the truck to respond to a head-on collision on Highway 520, a narrow, two-lane road notorious for its colossal wrecks and inevitable fatalities. I didn't sleep on this trip.

We happened to fall in behind one of the responding battalion chiefs, so we drove east in a speeding, two-vehicle convoy toward the river. The response seemed particularly long that night and we listened to the county's radio channel for a hint as to what to expect when we arrived. It couldn't have prepared us.

We arrived at the wreck and it looked like a staged scene of devastation. There was a light haze of smoke suspended above the mangled vehicles, the red pulsating lights from the emergency units flashing like beacons across the narrow road. The cars were lit by large spotlights that enhanced the wreckage, every metallic fold visible. The larger vehicle, a jacked-up pickup truck with oversized wheels, was lying on its side beside the roadway. A short distance away was a smaller vehicle, still sitting in the center of the road where it had been struck. Three drunken teenagers had crawled from the truck after it ran over the smaller car, which we later realized had been a convertible BMW. It was hard to tell at the time, since all that remained was the crushed remnant of the car with two dead bodies reclining in the front seats. The seats had been forced flat and the victims looked as if they had dozed off, only with crushing injuries to their heads and torsos from the weight of the speeding truck.

Apparently, the inebriated teens had been on their way back from the races that were held on an isolated dirt track near the county line. The races were notorious for their rowdy crowds and drunken fights. The teens' condition was no surprise to anyone. They belligerently argued with the officers, denying their intoxication as they stumbled over their words. Meanwhile, we stood by the BMW, each of us taking in the magnitude of the wreck, wondering about the people inside: who they were, where they were going, who they left behind. Realizing there were no patients to treat and that the police would take care of the teenagers, we loaded our equipment onto our stretcher and headed back to our truck. As George pulled away from the scene, I laid my head back and fell asleep as shadows of the wreck played against the background of my subconscious.

ALONE IN THE WOODS

For a year, I worked for a county ambulance service in a rural area of Tennessee north of Nashville. The relocation took place early in my career with OFD; I mention it now because of the similarity of working on an ambulance, yet in a very different setting. I would return to OFD shortly after.

It was a whole new world for me. I had been trained among the pampered emergency services of central Florida, where you have an abundance of personnel and close proximity to emergency rooms. I was not used to the isolation of a rural service, nor the distances you had to travel to reach an ER. It's amazing how fast a patient can crash when you are by yourself in the back of an ambulance with another thirty miles to cover before arriving at the hospital. At times, patient care was reduced to keeping the patient somewhat stable, hoping for the best, all the while urging your driver to haul ass.

Another difference between the metropolitan system of Orlando and the rural systems of Tennessee concerned the transportation of dead bodies. In Orlando, we didn't do it. When you had a death in the field, one in which the patient was so far gone that rigor mortis or decomposition had set in or the magnitude of trauma prevented any chance at resuscitation, you merely notified the police. They in turn notified the medical examiner, who then hauled away whatever remained of your patient. Robertson County, Tennessee, followed a different set of guidelines. I found this out the hard way, late one summer night when we were called out into the middle of the woods for a suicide.

We arrived at the scene, making our way down a narrow, worn-out dirt trail. The ambulance rocked wildly with each rut in the road as the police guided us in by radio. We pulled into a clearing and the only lights were the flashing red and whites from the patrol units. Their vehicles were arranged so their spotlights shone onto the lone car parked in the center of the small field, as if surrounding it for an ambush. It was an older black muscle car, the kind driven by young teenage boys who race through town, their tanned arms hanging out the window as they lean back smoking a cigarette. It's all part of an effect.

But this boy had given up on the effect, either through lack of success or boredom from trying. In fact, he had given up on everything. He had driven himself into the middle of the woods, rigged a hose from the exhaust pipe into the driver-side window, closed up the vehicle, and sprawled across the back seat. Perhaps the exhaust was not producing the anticipated effects, for he had also removed his belt from his faded denims and secured it tightly around his throat. The combined efforts had proven successful. He was quite dead when finally discovered by bystanders, who happened to spot his car after a long day of hunting.

The belt around his neck had caused the blood to pool in his face, which was black and bloated from the heat of the day. The rest of his body was slender and pliable and my partner and I had little trouble sliding him into the awaiting body bag. That was the first time I had ever seen or used a body bag, but it served its purpose quite well. We loaded him into the ambulance and drove out of the clearing. It was a strange feeling to be in the front seat with my partner, yet have a patient in the back of the truck with no one attending him. I kept glancing back into the dark compartment, certain I would see the body bag sit up on the stretcher and unzip itself. The experience was unsettling, and my partner couldn't drive fast enough.

We arrived at the hospital. The emergency room staff seemed perplexed that we would bring them a dead body. Somehow, there was some confusion as to protocol for the dead. The charge nurse shrugged, directing us to wheel him into the back hallway. There we located a stretcher and eased his slight frame onto the bed. As we left, I glanced back at the lone black bag in the empty hallway. He had died alone in the woods and now his body was being left in a back hallway. Every aspect of the incident magnified the isolation surrounding his death, and I couldn't help but wonder how long it would take for someone to claim him.

ASSAULTS

EMS CAN BE A THANKLESS JOB, PARTICULARLY WHEN THE PATIENTS take out their aggression on the rescuer. I happened to be on the receiving end on several occasions, but fortunately, most of the incidents were humorous rather than dangerous.

The humorous incidents usually involved drunks who decided they had had enough of our questions and would flail their arms in an attempt to land a punch. These were usually easy to escape. By the time the patient decided to fight, he typically lacked the ability to aim. Many times we would simply subdue the patient by strapping him down onto the stretcher and transporting him to the hospital, where he would spend the next few hours sleeping soundly as the ER buzzed around him.

One woman, an elderly diabetic, took a particular disliking to me as I tried to lift her from her chair to place her on the stretcher. She struck out, landing a surprisingly hearty slap to the right side of my face. I looked at her in astonishment as she smiled up at me, pleased with her aim. We wrestled her into the ambulance and as I bent over her to start an IV, she swung again. Her hand landed in the same spot as her first strike. At this point she was downright giddy with pride from her accuracy. From that point on, I kept one eye on her as I worked to stabilize her blood sugar. We transported her to the ER without further incidence, but I warned the hospital as we left her in its care.

Some of the assailants weren't even human. My partner and I had responded to a rural trailer located within the hills of Tennessee. Several tornados had touched down in the county, and we had spent most of the afternoon huddled around the radio, listening to weather updates, wondering where we would be called to next. Our patient had the audacity to call us out in the middle of the storm because her back had been hurting for several days. Why patients wait for the worst weather or the wee hours of the morning to report conditions that have been ongoing for days is one of the mysteries of EMS.

We pulled up in front of the shabby trailer and made our way around to the back. She had instructed the 911 operator that we were to enter her home through the back door. She probably hoped this would prevent us from trampling mud through her already filthy house. We assessed her, patiently listening to her litany of complaints and various medical disorders. We then loaded her onto our stretcher for transport. She told me her medications were in the back bedroom, so I made my way down the dark, narrow hallway to her room. Suddenly, there was a white flash at my feet. It grabbed onto my leg, driving its tiny teeth into the skin of my shin. Before I could kick free, the white flash was gone, having run from the room. It turned out to be a tiny white poodle, the kind that overcompensates for small stature with particular ferocity. I grabbed the bottles of medicine and was making my way back down the narrow hall when he struck again. The little beast had grabbed hold, this time nipping my ankle before high-tailing it back to the living room.

As I loaded her into the back of the ambulance, grumbling under my breath, the woman assured me the dog had all its shots. It was too comical to get seriously angry about. I cleaned the small wounds and shook off the incident.

I am fortunate to never have been seriously injured by a patient. But one incident reminded me that danger comes in many forms. Even in the form of small, quiet females.

We had been called out on a Saturday afternoon to a small two-story apartment. The caller had complained that her daughter, who had a serious psychiatric history, would not open the bedroom door and she was worried about her condition. We arrived on scene, accompanied by several police officers, and made our way up the narrow stairs to a locked bedroom. After no response from inside, the officers forced open the door. Inside we found a small teenage girl sitting on the floor under a window. The officers stepped aside as we entered the bedroom. My partner was holding the clipboard; I was carrying our jump bag. As we began to question the girl, I scanned the room. My partner continued to question her as I located several bottles of medicine on a small dresser.

I reached for the medicines, reading the labels of familiar antipsychotic meds as I turned to face my partner. Suddenly, I was struck on the forehead by a small yet sturdy fist. I stumbled backward, looking up in time to see the girl rush back to her spot under the window and bury her head in her folded arms. My partner and I were both stunned by her speed as I mechanically reached for my radio to call for backup. Although not seriously injured, all I could think about was what could have happened had she had a knife. She would have made an easy job of cutting my throat or plunging it into my chest, since my partner and I were distracted by our tasks.

From that point on I never took my eyes off psych patients, no matter how small or frail. A human being can move with incredible speed, especially fueled by anger and anxiety. Her family later informed me that the girl had forbidden anyone to touch her medicine. It would have been nice to have been given that tidbit of information upon our arrival.

A SLOW SATURDAY

It was one of my last shifts on the ambulance prior to beginning my career with OFD and the day was dragging. Sometimes it's hard to fill the hours of a slow shift, especially if they fall on a weekend when the pace of the city is diminished. The hours simply creep by. It was one of those long Saturday afternoons. George and I were busying ourselves by chatting with the ER staff about recent patients, new drug therapies, and exchanging the latest hospital gossip.

We were called out to the far edge of the county for an amputated toe. Thankful for a call to break up our boredom, we jumped into our unit and headed to the outskirts of our territory. Since the call was a long way out, the fire department decided to transport the patient instead of waiting for us. Our response was canceled and we returned to the emergency room to await their arrival.

The firefighters arrived, wheeling in a large, intoxicated man who seemed unconcerned that his Saturday was being interrupted by a trip to the ER. His left foot was wrapped in heavy white bandages. The same leg was bound in a dirty cast, obviously the result of some previous intoxicated mishap in which he sustained a fracture. He laughed loudly as they wheeled him into the examining room. The firefighters looked on with mild amusement as we followed them into the room.

The large dressings were removed, exposing the partially cast foot where a full set of toes used to be. Now, in place of the big toe, all that existed was a ground-down stub; only half of the second toe remained. I wracked my brain as to how this individual could have had the misfortune of amputating toes on a leg that was already damaged. Smiles danced across the faces of the firefighters as they repeated the story given to them upon arrival.

The man had fractured his lower leg several weeks prior. The details of this incident are too hazy to pull from my memory, but he inevitably suffered nerve damage, which diminished feeling in his foot. After several beers, he had decided it would be a great idea to go for a ride on the back of his friend's motorcycle. He had limped over, hopped on the back of the bike, and he and his friend had driven for several miles through the countryside. He was enjoying the ride when he happened to look down and noticed something wasn't right. He had a strange sensation in his foot so he tapped his friend on the shoulder and had him pull over. He was amazed to find he had two fewer toes than when he began the ride. Apparently he hadn't realized that his foot has slipped from the small pedal located on the rear wheel that serves as a resting place for the feet of passengers. Had they retraced their path, they would have found an interesting trail, for he had inadvertently been dragging the maimed leg on the cement, thereby grinding off his first and part of his second toe.

The emergency room staff proceeded to clean the wound, sewing together what remained of the former toes as they shook their heads in disbelief. The patient laughed and exchanged stories with the nurses. We had him to thank for breaking up what would have been a rather dull shift.

PART TWO

OFD

ROOKIE

About a year after becoming a medic I was hired by OFD. I was among twelve candidates who completed a two-week orientation during which we were taught rules and regulations and OFD fire-ground tactics. At the end of the two-week period, we anxiously awaited our assignments. I had already told anyone who would listen that I wanted to be assigned to Station 2. Why in the world I would ever want to work Station 2, with its all-nighters and heavy load of homeless people, was beyond my superiors, but I couldn't picture working anywhere else. I had spent the majority of my paramedic clinicals riding on Rescue 2. By the time I completed school the station had begun to feel like home. On the final day of orientation, we met for a formal lunch with the department's top administration. Following lunch, we lined up as our station assignments were read aloud. I held my breath as my assignment was announced: "Rescue 2, C Shift."

Station 2 was notorious for its call load. Sleep was a rare occurrence, the clientele were less than desirable, and HIV and TB patients accounted for a large majority of the patients. I, however, was eager for as much action as I could get. Shootings and stabbings were a regular occurrence in 2's territory and I thrived on trauma. To me, it was the most fascinating type of emergency call. Trauma patients are like puzzles needing to be put back together; it's never the same combination of injuries. Gunshot wounds involving various parts of the body, multisystem traumas from high-speed collisions, or beatings resulting in massive blunt-force trauma: such patients require lightning-fast decisions and immediate action. The pace is exhilarating.

I was not disappointed. I worked numerous traumas during my time on Rescue 2, becoming well versed in trauma protocol and honing my skills in patient assessment. I became used to the frenetic pace and lack of sleep. I came to know the west side of town, an area I never knew existed before entering the field of EMS. Growing up in a middle-class neighborhood, I was oblivious to the poverty that existed just west of downtown. I became fascinated with the people: the way they lived, the way they eked out an existence. I came to know the regulars, those with medical conditions requiring regular attention. We would assess them, try to make them comfortable, and send them on to the hospital when necessary. Many of the residents were kind and appreciative. They had watched over the years as their neighborhoods deteriorated and the drug dealers moved in. They played silent witness to the increase in violence and the proliferation of the homeless. Still, they maintained their small homes, holding fast to their version of the American dream.

Station 2 housed a rescue truck, a fire engine, and a ladder truck. Two personnel were assigned to the rescue; three or four personnel rode the engine (depending on manning), and the ladder required four. "Engineers" were responsible for driving and operating each truck. The rescue was assigned an engineer and firefighter, both of whom were paramedics. The engine was assigned an engineer, a lieutenant (who was in charge of the unit), and at least one firefighter. The truck was assigned an engineer, lieutenant, and two firefighters. The lieutenants were also in charge of the station itself, and the rescue fell under the direction of the ladder truck officer.

OFD utilizes rigid standard operating procedures (SOPs) on all emergency scenes. The SOPs are based on a "split team" concept, where personnel from each truck have clearly defined duties and tasks on emergency scenes. For instance, on a typical house fire, the engine crew's sole responsibility is to advance a hose line, locate the seat of the fire, and extinguish the blaze. The rescue personnel are split between the tower team; the engineer works with the "outside team" from the tower truck and the other medic works with the "inside team." The outside team's responsibilities include ventilating the structure, placing ladders into windows for the evacuation of victims and the escape of personnel, and ventilating the roof when necessary. The inside team's responsibilities include search and rescue, ventilation, and assisting the engine crew.

Everything happens in concert on a fire scene. The rapid completion of tasks is fundamental to controlling the scene, and it's thrilling to watch crews descend on a fire and bring it under control. As each objective is met, the officer in charge of the scene relays the information to Dispatch in the form of verbal "benchmarks." These include "water on the fire," "all clear" (when the search for victims is complete), and "fire knocked down" (when the main body of the fire is under control).

Daily station duties are completed by all crew members. Chores are divided among personnel and rotate each month. The engineers oversee the firefighters and the lieutenants oversee everyone. My lieutenants at Station 2 were seasoned veterans, each with nearly twenty years on the department. They were "salty," meaning they had amassed a career's worth of experience and were well versed in fighting fire. They were still becoming accustomed to females on the department. I was only the eighth female hired in the history of the department, so the majority of crews had yet to have a female assigned to their stations. My orientation to the station consisted of one of the lieutenants sitting me down in the office, eyeing me suspiciously, and saying "On a fire scene, you're assigned to the truck, but basically you're on your own." That was it. No insight into the inner workings of crews. No words of wisdom or advice. Yes, I had completed orientation with the other new hires, which included OFD's standard operating procedures, but I was hoping for some form of guidance, some direction to navigating among my fellow firefighters. I quickly realized I was definitely on my own and concentrated on fitting in with my new crew.

FIRST NIGHT

My first night at Station 2 will forever live on in my memory, but not for the number of calls, the number of lives saved, or the size of the fires. It lives on in my memory as a night of fear: fear of the dreaded alert buzzer. I had become acquainted with the buzzer while a student and in that short time had come to loathe it. It was a jarring, excruciatingly loud alarm that would rattle your teeth if you happened to be standing under it when a call came in.

As my years on the department grew in number, many aspects of the field evolved to better accommodate those performing the job. Equipment became lighter, hoses became more flexible, and the alert tones within our stations became more listener-friendly. But I was hired prior to many of these advances. Therefore, my first night was spent in anticipation of what I knew to be a gut-wrenching alert tone designed to scare the shit out of anyone who had the nerve to think he was going to get a few hours of sleep. The fact that I was assigned to the busiest truck in the city didn't help matters. The calls were inevitable.

I had spent nights at a fire station before. But the quiet station in Maitland was located in an upper-class area and the call loads were relatively light. The chances of calls in the middle of the night were scarce and the station was designed for comfort, not the fierce efficiency required by Orlando's west side. The stations of the west side were fortified structures designed for rapid response times. Most of the nights were spent sliding the pole to respond and climbing the stairs back to bed. Such was the case at Station 2.

I knew what to expect that first night. But the calls were not the only thing keeping me wide-eyed throughout the night. The dorm itself didn't help matters. Prior to the politically correct design of new fire stations, the dorms of older stations were designed for one thing: to house as many bunks as possible in as little space necessary.

Sleeping in a large room with a bunch of men can be a bit intimidating. The closeness of their bunks took some getting used to, and there were many nights where I would lie awake, fantasizing about strangling the firefighter at the other end of the room who persistently snored loud enough to rattle the windows. Aside from the strangeness of the surroundings, the thermostat was kept at a crisp fifty degrees and I would curl up in a tight ball and still wake up with numb extremities. I never understood the reasoning behind such cold dorms. Later on, when I had some time under my belt and a few rookies beneath me, I would casually walk by the thermostat on my way back to bed and give it a hefty nudge into the sixties.

So my first night was spent waiting for the deafening tone that, as luck would have it, didn't come until around 5:00 A.M. By that time I was practically in a trance from staring at the ceiling all night and don't remember the nature of the call or even if I killed the patient. Over the years, I eventually learned to tolerate being repeatedly jolted out of bed, but I can't say that I miss it.

DELIVERY

One of the few positive events for which emergency personnel are called is childbirth. The delivery of a child is fairly straightforward. In some cultures, the expectant mother, heavy with impending birth, makes her way alone to a birthing hut. There she squats in a small woven hammock especially designed for the event, delivering the infant alone. She then cuts the cord with a rudimentary knife made of local stone, wiping the mucus from the baby's mouth and placing it gently to her breast. My first delivery was not quite as simple.

My partner and I were called to a small house several blocks from the station. Many of the houses are small wood-frame structures with uneven floors and deteriorating porches. We followed the cries of our patient into a tiny back bedroom, crammed with secondhand furniture and smelling of old ashtrays and sweat. The patient was lying on her back, legs bent, uncaring that she greeted us with her bulging genitalia. The baby's head was crowning, signaling its impending birth.

My partner, a veteran with several deliveries under his belt, calmly handed me the obstetrics kit and said in his low, gruff tone "This one's yours." As steadily as I could, I threw open the kit, laying out the equipment I would need, all the while aware of the small head that kept easing outward with each contraction. The mother was young, black, and had that intense look of determination new mothers have as they try to free their bodies from the small passenger they have been toting around for nine months. I spoke to her in quiet but directing tones, telling her to continue to pant. I quickly donned sterile gloves and slid a surgical pad under her buttocks, something clean to catch the baby in case I failed.

I placed a gentle gloved hand on the head of the infant and could feel its slimy texture and the force of the mother's body as it tried to expel it. With a final push, the head came forth and a small pinched face appeared. I guided its rotation and began suctioning its nose and mouth. The baby was a strange purplish-blue, like an eggplant that had been cooked a bit too long. I watched as it made silent progress from the mother's body. As the shoulders emerged, I could see the pulsing umbilical cord wrapped tightly around its small neck. I slid my fingers beneath the cord, frantically trying to loosen it enough to slip it over the small head. As the shoulders delivered, the rest of the body quickly followed. I balanced the baby's weight in one hand as I forced my hand between its shoulder blades, up and under the constricting band. I remember thinking how ironic it was that the source of life for the baby for nine months might just be the cause of its demise if I didn't get it from around his throat. With the baby delivered, the cord slackened enough that I could slip it over the small head. I quickly inverted the infant across by palm, trying to stimulate it to breathe. Its limp legs straddled my wrist. As I suctioned its airway, I aggravated it enough that it started breathing on its own. It kicked its tiny purple legs and began to sputter and wail.

The little eggplant had sprung to life and I watched in amazement as its purple skin faded to the normal mottled tone of newborns. The young mother laid back in sweaty relief, her eyes never leaving the small form. I wiped it clean, wrapped it in aluminum foil to maintain its body heat, and placed it on the mother's chest. She looked like a young girl clutching an oversized baked potato. We loaded her into the ambulance and I carried the little potato at my chest. I smiled with pride as the small metallic bundle grimaced the whole way to the hospital. I reluctantly turned it over to the awaiting obstetrics team and made my way out into the warm night.

MAN DOWN

Halloween always makes for an interesting shift. Typically crews spend the evening chasing dumpster fires started by bored kids who have outgrown trick-or-treating, yet are too young to get into the drunken street parties held downtown.

We had spent the day carving a large pumpkin to place in front of the station, a pumpkin that would invariably end up smashed on the front sidewalk when the young hoodlums were too tired to locate another dumpster. But we carved it anyway, if only to have the seeds to bake for a late snack in between the burning containers of trash.

We had the usual procession of costumed children, guided by parents who knew one of the few safe places to obtain candy from strangers is at the local fire station. We took turns donning a grotesque mask and hiding in the bushes near the front of the station. We would jump out at the trick-or-treaters, scaring the shit out of them as they timidly approached our doors. Firefighters are, by all accounts, good-natured humanitarians as well as devilish pranksters.

The evening was growing late, the dumpsters mundane, when we received a call for a "man down" on the East/West Expressway. Further details en route stated the victim was a possible auto-versus-pedestrian. Our Halloween was about to turn bloody. Anyone hit by the high-speed vehicles that traverse the expressway would surely be categorized as severe trauma. We rushed to the scene with sirens screaming.

Traffic had slowed in the area and we wove in between cars that couldn't decide whether to move aside or ease forward for a better look. The victim lay face down, dressed in jeans and an oversized flannel shirt. A floppy hat was perched on his head, and I was amazed that a person could withstand a high-speed impact and yet retain his accessories. In fact, there was no blood, no tissue, no pool of bodily fluids that typically accompany an auto-versus-pedestrian at high speed. We jumped from the truck and grabbed our medical bags, backboard, and cervical collar, certain we would need them to package what remained of the individual. We approached with caution, since even trauma victims can come up swinging. I tapped his foot and called out to him. No response. We crouched down to gingerly feel for a pulse when we noticed he had heavy gloves on his hands. In fact, every inch of his body was covered, leaving no skin exposed. As we gently prodded him for signs of life, we noticed that the trunk of his body was curiously fluffy. Realizing we had been duped, we flung him onto his back, revealing a human form stuffed with hay. Laughing in relief, we loaded our scarecrow onto the back of the truck. There he sat, propped up and smiling, as he accompanied us back to the station.

DESPERATION

THEY SAY IN CENTRAL FLORIDA YOU CAN'T TRAVEL MORE THAN A MILE without encountering a body of water. This doesn't include the thousands of swimming pools, which look like small, blue jewels glistening in the sun when you travel by air. Thus, it amazes me that I have only been to one drowning in my thirteen years as a medic in Florida.

He was an overweight man in his forties. He had been staying at a crummy hotel in one of the worst sections of Orlando. He was probably one step from landing in the homeless shelter, using his few remaining dollars for a dingy bed and a fading sense of self-sufficiency. After a heavy night of drinking in which he probably agonized over his current financial situation, he wandered onto the back lot of the hotel where a low metal fence encircled a grimy pool and a murky Jacuzzi. He chose the Jacuzzi. He eased his weight into the bubbling froth, clothed only in his underwear, still clutching his bottle. Perhaps he wanted to die. Perhaps he planned to drink himself into a stupor and slide beneath the churning water. That's exactly what happened.

We arrived to find that a few bystanders had managed to drag his lifeless form from the water. As we worked on him, I thought about his last moments, floating in the water until someone happened to pass by and notice. I pictured the hesitant bystanders, nervously milling around after discovering him, the smarter one choosing to run to the front office for help, the others left staring at each other, wondering who should be the first in the water, the first to check for signs of life, the first to grab hold of the victim.

He didn't make it. The majority of drownings are better off dying. In the rare case when a pulse is restored, the families are usually left with a severely brain-damaged individual whom they must now feed and change or visit at a nursing home. Most of the time death is better.

SUDDENLY

Some of the most disturbing calls are those in which the individual is killed instantly. To stand over a body that was, moments before, alive with thoughts, fears, and plans can truly fuck with your head. All that the person once was is now replaced by a vacant emptiness that settles in the pupils following death. These are the calls that burrow into my subconscious, peeking out at the most inopportune moments. Like when I am laughing with friends or trying to fall back to sleep at 3:00 A.M.

Each time I was called to these scenes, I knew what was to follow. We would discreetly cover the body to shield it from curious onlookers, and to escape the blank stares of the dead as we stood by, impotent and silent. We would mill around, kicking debris from the roadway, waiting for the arrival of the medical examiner's technicians: those poor guys that gather the remains of the dead, neatly packaging them for transport to the cold, metallic tables of the city morgue.

Several of these calls stand out in my mind, ones that were particularly haunting. Like the boy we found several hours after his car had left the roadway and flipped into a ditch. He had been pinned under the vehicle, under the shallow, murky water of recent rains. The only visible sign of him had been a small pale foot protruding from beneath the surface.

Or the young girl who had sped into the night following a fight with her boyfriend, only to slam her car into the back end of a slow-moving street sweeper she hadn't seen as she wiped the tears of frustration from her face. The boyfriend, concerned for her safety, had followed, only to come upon the wreck and find her crumpled against the steering wheel, her body broken and still.

Or the middle-aged man who was driving his van through a residential street, only to be struck broadside by another vehicle. As the top-heavy van turned onto its side, the unrestrained driver came out of his seat and through the open window, the van landing on his head with a muffled crunch. We found the remains of his brain and large pieces of skull several feet away in the gutter, as onlookers held one hand to their mouths and pointed with the other. But the most disturbing aspect was the unanswered ringing of his car phone. I still think about this scene when I try to reach a loved one and can't.

These calls have a way of merging into one long, silent movie. They flash before my mind's eye in grainy black and white, yet I see each scene in fine detail. I hear the sounds that accompanied each call: the splashing of boots in water, the ping of cooling metal. The smells return: those of spilled oil, battery acid, and blood. And as my mind rebuilds each scene, the healthier segment of my subconscious tears them down, replacing them with kinder memories of my years in EMS.

THE CATCH

I'VE DELIVERED FOUR BABIES IN MY YEARS ON THE JOB. FORTUNATELY, all have been screaming and kicking by the time I was through with them. I was happy to retire with a perfect track record. Most of them went relatively smoothly. One of them I was barely in time for, and the mother delivered on the front seat of her car as I approached the vehicle. I managed to wrap the baby and cut the cord as she and her husband laughed and wept.

Another I delivered in a hotel room, where a very large woman quickly delivered her fourth child. I barely had time to glove up when the latest edition to the family arrived at the Holiday Inn. We eventually had to load her onto a backboard and ease her out onto the bucket of our ladder truck, since the railing outside her second-story room did not provide enough space to maneuver her large frame around the corner. The truck company was only too happy to assist, since they rarely got the opportunity to attend births. But my last field delivery will always stick in my mind as a moment of sheer panic.

We were called to an upstairs apartment in one of the small, block-construction buildings downtown. It was early morning and the young patient, around seventeen years of age, was there with both parents, a rarity for that part of town, where single-parent homes were the norm. The parents were in good humor, perhaps focusing on the event at hand and not the future responsibility of having an additional mouth to feed. They chatted happily as I assessed the girl. Although she was full term, her contractions had just started and her water had yet to break. We had plenty of time.

She kept complaining of "feeling something down there," pointing to her pubic region. I asked her if it felt as if she needed to move her bowels, since this is a common sensation of mothers on the verge of delivery. She agreed and we prepped her for the arrival of the ambulance that would take her to the hospital. As I heard the ambulance approach, I instructed her that we would slowly walk her out of the apartment and toward the outer stairway. Due to the narrowness of the outer balcony, the ambulance would set up a stretcher at the base of the stairs. I thought the brief walk might do her some good, since her contractions didn't seem to be progressing.

I led her out. She was clothed in nothing but a sheer, knee-length nightgown. The ambulance personnel were walking toward the stairs with their stretcher as I eased her along the balcony. The walkway was rather long and at one point, she complained about the sensation again of "something down there." I decided to take a peak, so I squatted down in front of her and lifted her gown. The walkway was completely dark, but there was a spotlight at the opposite end of the balcony. Her body presented in silhouette and I'll never forget what I saw. Suspended in her underwear hung the large head of a newborn.

I saw my career flash before my eyes. I could see the headlines: "Paramedic lets baby fall to concrete! Story on page 2." I ordered her to immediately lie down and called down to the ambulance personnel to bring me a light ASAP, since our end of the walkway was cloaked in darkness. I ripped off her underwear and managed to get a hand under the head of the infant just as the rest of the baby slid from her body. I felt around the neck for the umbilical cord, all the while juggling the slimy little critter between my hands, unable to see a thing. The medics bounded up the stairs with a light as the infant began to wail, reassuring me that it was trying its best to cooperate and that my career might not be over after all.

The baby and mother were fine. My heart rate eventually dropped below 200 as we loaded her into the ambulance for transport. I could never figure out how she was able to deliver so quickly. Perhaps her water had broken when she was on the toilet earlier and she just didn't notice. Perhaps she had an oversized birth canal that enabled a supersonic delivery. Perhaps it was just a bizarre incident that will live on in EMS infamy. I don't know. All I know is that from that point on, I never took anything for granted when it came to deliveries in the field.

THE INFANT

When you think of Florida, you generally envision clear skies and the intensity of a tropical sun. One rarely thinks of fog. But during certain times of the year, when the cool air of morning meets the warmth of the earth and the humidity rises, a dense fog can settle on the land, even among the crowded streets of downtown.

It was one of those mornings, when the fog had formed while we slept through a strangely quiet Saturday night. When the tones went off early the next morning, summoning us to an "infant not breathing," we rubbed the sleep from our eyes as we made our way to our trucks.

When you get called to an infant not breathing, it usually turns out to be one of two things: either a new parent has panicked over the erratic belly-breathing of their newborn, or a baby has died of SIDS. I had a feeling this one was going to be the latter. The timing was classic: early in the morning, the mother perhaps noticing how strangely quiet her night had been. She wanders in to check on the baby whom she believes has just made it through their first night without crying. What she finds will forever change her.

We pulled out of the station and the fog encircled us. The lights flashing from our trucks played against it, casting eerie shadows as we wove through the crumbling neighborhoods of our territory. We pulled up to the scene and I jumped from the truck. I grabbed the airway bag and ran into the house to get a quick head start on patient care.

When I entered the house I was amazed by two things: the tightness of the tiny rooms and the number of individuals residing within. There were people everywhere. They must have had at least nine people living in that small, two-bedroom house, ranging in age from toddlers to the elderly; several generations represented. Someone in a back bedroom was screaming, so I followed the sound into a dim room that contained several beds surrounded by piles of clothes. There were a lot people in the room, all surrounding the woman I assumed to be the mother of the infant since she was making the most noise. As she cried out, she pointed to a lower bunk bed where a small form lay. I crouched down and my initial impression was of a doll. The baby didn't appear real or alive. It was incredibly small, lying motionless in a dirty pink sleeper.

When we approach patients with no vital signs and are unsure how long they have been "down," we go for the jaw. Rigor mortis sets into the muscles of the jaw first, so it is usually an efficient guide in determining whether you should begin CPR or make other arrangements. I grabbed the baby's small chin. It was firm and stiff. As the rest of my crew entered the room, I subtly shook my head. They backed out of the room in silence. I now had to explain things to the mother.

I typically found it was easier to focus on the mechanics of such calls: first, explain that the patient has been dead too long for resuscitative measures to be effective; next, let the family know that the police were responding and that they would see to the arrangements from this point on; and finally, offer any type of assistance, such as talking to family or simply staying on scene a while to offer support. As I went through the process with the mother, she continued to wail and claw at my arms. I tried to comfort her while avoiding looking at the baby. The relatives finally led her from the room and I stayed behind to find a blanket to cover the child. It was at this point I finally took a good look at it.

It was so small. It must have been premature and perhaps had even spent time in one of the cozy plastic incubators of the neonate unit. But this baby had other problems aside from its size. Somewhere in the developmental process, something had gone wrong. Perhaps through some genetic hiccup or the use of crack cocaine so popular in this part of town, the stage during which the hands and feet developed had been skipped. The baby was left with small clubs where those elements should have been. It never had a chance. I covered the small form with a cotton blanket, arranging it with the cleanest side down and tucking it around those tiny deformed limbs before silently leaving the room.

We walked toward our trucks. The quiet of the morning, mixed with the heaviness of the fog, lent a surreal aspect to our surroundings. The parking lights of the police cars were small points of light as we eased our trucks from between them, heading back to the station.

THE BURNING ROOM

I have only been to one house fire that involved the death of an infant. The fire occurred late at night, on one of those rare, frigidly cold winter nights in Florida. We were called to the scene after the fact. The first-arriving trucks had already put out the fire. We were there to "overhaul" the scene, which meant searching for burning embers and shoveling debris. The scene was lit by the powerful spotlights of our trucks, and the investigators carefully worked among the remains of what had previously been the small, cozy residence of an elderly couple and their infant grandchild. The lingering warmth of the fire mixed with the cold night air, casting a steamy haze over the scene. Our personnel moved like ghosts among the burned-out structure, and the pungent taste of smoldering debris settled in our mouths.

The house had been cold that night, like most of the wood-framed homes in the area lacking central heat. So the grandfather had plugged in the aging space heater, moving it close to the baby, who had been sleeping in the living room on a makeshift bed. But it had done more than warm the child. It had radiated enough heat to catch the worn-out drapes covering the windows on fire, quickly spreading through the small room. The grandfather had awakened to the noise of the fire, but instead of grabbing the baby and running to safety, he had chosen to go outside for the garden hose in an attempt to extinguish the blaze.

A garden hose is no match for a house fire. Fire can consume a wooden structure with frightening speed. He soon realized the house and baby were lost, as he ran back and forth in front of the structure with his hands held to his head in desperation and shock. The grandparents had been taken to the hospital for treatment for burns they sustained trying to rescue the infant. Now the scene was left to us.

We were sent to the rear of the house to shovel out what remained of the charred contents. This included clothing, the remains of a small bed, and the burned remnants of furniture. While I dug into the closet, I scooped out a small, clear jar that contained a large roll of bills. I assumed it was their life's savings, tucked safely in the back of the closet behind old clothes and photo albums. I turned it over to the police, wondering if that small jar of money was the last of their possessions, all that remained of a life spent in hard labor bent over a mop or working in the heat of a factory.

We finished with the back of the house and I made my way around to the front of the structure, peering inside at the blackened remnants of their home. The investigators had placed spotlights in the front room to provide lighting for the medical examiner to photograph the infant. What remained of the child was unrecognizable. All that was left was the deeply charred torso, which resembled a small chicken breast that someone had forgotten on the barbeque. The investigators spoke in the quiet tones reserved for scenes of death as the last of the neighbors mingled across the street, murmuring and shaking their heads.

We continued working in the cold, picking up the last of their lives and making a neat pile of their ruined belongings. I wondered to myself where they would begin in the morning. We gratefully returned to the warmth of our station as the first hints of daylight broke in the eastern sky.

UNDER THE CAMPER

THERE ARE FOUR WORDS ON A FIRE SCENE THAT CAN STOP PARAMEDICS in their tracks: "We have a victim." For a paramedic, those words signify a shift from firefighting activities to those of patient care and are usually accompanied by disappointment and disgruntled cursing. The opportunity to fight fire is a rare occurrence; patient care is the mainstay of EMS. To have the adrenaline-pumping activities of firefighting interrupted by someone complaining of smoke inhalation is rather deflating. Such was the case on a hot afternoon when we responded to a large auto repair shop for a commercial building fire.

At the time, I was assigned to Rescue 1, the city's large, heavy rescue truck. Rescue 1 is equipped with specialized extrication tools, from hydraulic spreaders and jacks that can take apart a vehicle to heavy-duty air bags that can lift a locomotive. Rescue 1 was part of the Special Teams housed at Station 1, along with the Dive Team, the Hazardous Materials Team, and the High Angle Rescue Team. It was a great assignment.

My partner and I pulled up on the scene, positioning our truck out of the way of the engines and ladder trucks yet close enough to enable the retrieval of equipment. As we climbed down from the cab, donning our air packs and gathering our tools, someone on scene delivered those fateful words: "We have a victim." I decided to leave my air pack on, just in case it turned out to be a minor complaint and I could still catch some fire. This would not be the case.

The structure was a long building composed of open bays where specially trained mechanics repaired large travel campers. The crews were directing their actions to the area of heavy smoke coming from one end of the building. As we approached the scene, equipment in hand, we found firefighters surrounding a severely burned young man standing upright in the middle of one of the bays. He had his arms extended in front of him, poised like a sleepwalker, yet his eyes were wide with fright. He was a boy of about eighteen and his skin, which had been black, now consisted of large white patches fringed with charred edges. Translucent sheets of skin hung in tatters from his body. His clothing had been burned off and all that remained were the soles of his tennis shoes and a small patch of material covering his groin. He didn't say a word, but his face had that blankness of someone who knows they are in deep shit.

We quickly placed a backboard on the ground and I ripped open a sterile burn sheet and spread it on the board. I gently took his hands, avoiding the thin layers of dangling flesh, and led him down onto the sheet. We wrapped him in additional sheets to prevent further contamination of his wounds and immediately loaded him for transport as one of his coworkers gave me a brief account of the incident.

The boy had been working under a camper at the far end of the building. He was trying to repair a leak in a fuel line when the line broke, dousing him in gasoline. He crawled out from under the camper and made his way through the bays toward a shower located at the far end of the building, trying to shake off the excess fuel, probably frustrated at his own clumsiness. As he proceeded through the open bays, another mechanic was busy using an acetylene torch. The boy apparently walked too close to the torch; its flying sparks found the vapors trailing the boy, igniting his trail and instantly setting him ablaze. He had run from his coworkers as they tried to douse the flames until they finally managed to hose him down.

As we rushed to the hospital, the ambulance medic notified the ER, advising them that we would be delivering a severely burned patient. The hospital assembled their burn team and prepared for our arrival. I placed oxygen on the boy and tried to assess his vital signs. The sterile sheets and condition of his skin prevented me from obtaining a blood pressure. I listened to his lungs and examined his airway for signs of inhalation burns. He began to speak in a surprisingly clear voice, asking me if he was going to make it.

This was the first severely burned patient I had ever worked on. I knew how to assess such a patient, but I had yet to understand the mechanics of severe burns. Because the boy was not having trouble breathing and the mucus membranes lining his respiratory track appeared healthy and pink, I thought he might have a chance. I spoke to him gently and shared the positive findings. I didn't know that with such severe burns the body reacts in frightening ways and that within hours, his 180-pound frame would swell to over 300 pounds due to severe edema of the tissues. He was dead by morning.

That call had come on the tail end of a long weekend. I had worked a double shift two days before, covering for one of my coworkers. During that time, I had worked three separate cardiac arrests: two of them elderly patients with cardiac histories, the third a young man in an auto accident. The auto accident had occurred early in the morning, on the expressway near one of the exit toll plazas. Apparently the young man was returning home following a midnight shift at one of Orlando's numerous hotels near Disney World. He must have dozed off, for his car continued at full speed until it found the back end of a semi that had rolled to a stop to pay the toll. He had slammed into the back of the tanker truck, which fortunately was only carrying milk. The impact had been so great that the seams along both legs of his pants had split when his legs crashed into the dash.

Ironically, the two previous cardiac arrests had both been saves. This boy didn't have a chance. The possibilities of reviving a patient following a traumatic cardiac arrest are practically nonexistent. But the frustration over such situations lingers and the anxiety associated with those calls can wear down the soul. I have often tried to add up the number of deaths I have witnessed on the job, but it's an impossible task. The numbers blur over time and all that remains are faint memories. I suppose this is the mind's way of smoothing the edges so that we can process and store them without reliving every detail. It's like taking a sharp object, wrapping it in cloth so it no longer cuts, and tucking it safely away in your pocket.

DEATH BY SUICIDE

SUICIDE COMES IN MANY FORMS. THEY EACH REEK OF ANGUISH, AND the patient is usually left in a condition no family member should ever have to witness. That's what amazes me about some suicides: their total disregard for the mess they leave behind. I have often wondered why people who kill themselves don't at least have the decency to leave behind a tidy corpse.

Many of the suicides I have been called to were extremely messy affairs. One of them, a prominent physician recently diagnosed with terminal cancer, at least had the forethought to go into the back shed of his lovely two-story house before putting a shotgun to his chest and blowing a hole through his torso. Another elderly patient, also recently diagnosed, also chose the shotgun, although he was thoughtful enough to sit in the bathtub prior to putting both barrels into his mouth. Still, he should have anticipated the mess his head would make. We were called to his small yellow house on a weekend afternoon. I was a firefighter assigned to Engine 5. The other firefighter was a rookie with only two shifts under his belt. We arrived on the scene and were greeted by a sheriff's deputy standing in the doorway. His large frame took up most of the space as he slowly shook his head, indicating the futility of the call.

He pointed to the back bathroom and I took my equipment and my rookie with me. I could see the nervousness in the rookie's eyes. He was about to get a strong dose of reality.

I entered the small bathroom and tried to take in the gruesomeness of the scene. The man was huddled in the bathtub. The shotgun still sat between his legs and the remains of his shattered head rested on lifeless shoulders. The left side of his face was gone and his right eye hung down from fibers still attached within the socket. I surveyed the small room, noting the splattering of tissue that had been sprayed across every surface. All I could think about was how difficult the mess would be to clean up and if his poor, elderly wife would ever be able to erase this image from her mind. She had been in the back room resting when the blast from the gun startled her from sleep. She had entered the bathroom, only to find the remains of her husband's head sprayed throughout the room, his body a mangled mess within the tub. I thought of all the neat ways in which someone can kill themselves, ways that would spare those left behind from such horrifying scenes. Suicides can be extremely self-centered.

I have been to too many suicides to accurately count. Their reasons are numerous, with impending terminal illness one of the most common. Another of the most dramatic cases for which we were called was not dispatched as a suicide at all. We responded to a "patient burned."

Although the call was outside the city limits, we responded mutual aid with the county due to our close proximity to the address. Because of the vagueness of the dispatch, we donned our gear in case active fire was involved. We pulled up to the scene of a small aging strip mall consisting of three businesses. There was a moderate amount of smoke coming from a store on one end, so we jumped from the truck anticipating a structure fire. But before we had a chance to pull a line from the engine, we were accosted by bystanders who screamed and pointed to the blanketed form lying in the parking lot.

Since I was the primary paramedic on the truck, I quickly shed my gear to attend to the patient. The rest of my crew continued into the structure to extinguish the blaze. I grabbed what equipment I could, instructing two bystanders to carry the rest. I approached the form on the ground, noting the smoldering blue blanket that covered him. I gently removed the blanket, finding a severely burned man in his midthirties. He was burned over 95 percent of his body, his face the only area not red or blackened. His arms were folded tightly across his chest and he stared straight into the sky, fully conscious. I tried to get him to speak, but he gazed passed me, ignoring my questions. There was blood seeping from both wrists. I spoke quietly, trying to get him to respond.

I wrapped him carefully, folding his charred body into sterile sheets. As the fire progressed, the smoke banked down, covering us in a dark, brown haze. The ambulance arrived and we gently lifted him onto the stretcher, slowly making our way through the dense cloud. I was able to extend his arms enough to start two large-bore intravenous lines in an attempt to hydrate his decimated body. Throughout the ride to the hospital, he never broke his silence. I found out later what had happened.

Having recently been diagnosed HIV positive, the patient had decided he would rather take his own life than have it slowly wrenched from him through the long, slow process of AIDS. He arrived at work that morning to the small shop where he designed stained glass. He had taken a knife and cut both wrists, but it had not had the desired effect. He then took the chemicals he used to create his beautiful windows and doused himself before lighting himself on fire. He had run from the shop in flames, leaving behind enough of the burning chemicals to catch the building on fire. He had made it to the parking lot where frightened bystanders had covered him with a blanket, finally smothering the flames.

Somehow he managed to survive for almost a month with his injuries. We continued to check on his progress until he finally succumbed to his injuries. I suppose he got what he wanted. What we got were the memories of his badly burned body and awards of commendation for our actions on the fire ground.

SPECIAL EFFECTS

It's a common occurrence for a call to turn out to be of a nature completely different from the original dispatch. Many times we responded to "cardiac" calls that turned out to be stomach disorders. "Accidents with entrapment" regularly turned out to be minor crashes with no one trapped. So when we received the call for a "self-inflicted stabbing to the chest" I naturally assumed it would turn out to be something else, like a sobbing teenager who had scratched herself for attention after downing a handful of Tylenol.

We pulled up to a well-manicured lawn as a woman in her fifties came rushing from the front door, screaming that her daughter had tried to kill herself again. As we carried our equipment inside, I began questioning the woman. Before the mother had a chance to explain, I arrived in her kitchen to find a young woman lying face up in the middle of the floor with a six-inch butcher knife sticking out of the center of her chest. She was pale and diaphoretic and I watched as the knife pulsated with each beat of her heart. It looked like a scene from a low-budget horror film, yet the wound was real and we had to act.

The primary objective in treating impaled objects is to stabilize them in place, thus minimizing damage to surrounding tissues and organs. This was going to be tricky. The woman was alive but unconscious. She had several smaller practice wounds on her upper abdomen, apparently inflicted before she decided to kneel on the kitchen floor and fall onto the knife to ensure penetration. She lay bare-chested on the floor, arms and legs spread eagle, with the black handle of the knife protruding just to the left of her breastbone. We quickly piled several trauma dressings around the handle, taping them in place and preparing for the inevitable cardiac arrest.

We loaded her into the ambulance, rapidly applying oxygen, cardiac monitor, and two large-bore intravenous lines to help maintain her blood pressure and pulse. When we arrived at the ER, we wheeled her into the trauma room as the hospital staff looked on in amazement. The trauma surgeons went to work, barking orders for equipment, tests, and for someone to find a camera.

They worked furiously on her, trying to assess the extent of her injury and the exact location of the tip of the knife. The x-ray revealed it was lying just alongside her heart, but had inevitably penetrated the surrounding vasculature, since she was rapidly bleeding out into her chest. They eventually performed one of the most dramatic procedures that can take place within an emergency room—cracking the chest. The surgeon makes an incision across the chest following the angle of the ribs, usually just below the nipple line. This allows full access to the internal organs and enables the surgeon to manually massage the heart in an attempt to circulate blood. The location of the incision will depend on the location of the injury. In her case, they opened up the entire chest, cutting through the breastbone, so that they could visualize the location of the knife in relation to her heart.

It didn't work. Once they had the chest opened, they were able to remove the knife, but by that time, she had slipped into irreversible shock. The large volumes of intravenous fluids used to initially boost her falling blood pressure could only sustain her for so long. These fluids are very effective for replacing blood volume but they lack one very important capability: the ability to transport oxygen. Patients with traumatic injuries accompanied by significant blood loss can be stabilized for a while, but eventually the body shuts down because of lack of oxygen to the tissues.

Her blood pressure stabilized briefly, but the rest of her body began to fail. We stood by watching the falling numbers on the cardiac monitor until the surgeons exhausted their protocols and called it quits. She was left on the table, her chest opened and her injured heart exposed. Beside her on a small metal table, among the bloodied surgical instruments, was the large black-handled knife.

THE BOY IN THE ROAD

It's strange, the things you remember most about a call. Sometimes it's an aspect of the call itself, like the time of day or season. Sometimes it's the nature of the call, particularly if it's traumatic. Other times it's an aspect of the patient's physical appearance, such as their height or weight, especially when those are extreme. For me, what stands out in my mind when I reflect on certain calls are the looks on the faces of my patients. The look of pain, frustration, fear, and desperation can leave lasting impressions. But sometimes it's the lack of human emotion that can haunt one's memory. Such is the case in severe head injuries.

It was a Sunday, late in the day. It had been relatively quiet; the call broke the calm of the afternoon. The call didn't come via Dispatch, but from a frantic bystander pounding on our station door saying a boy had been struck by a car down the street. We jumped into the engine and drove the short distance down the street where a young blond boy was sprawled face up in the middle of the roadway. We grabbed our medical bags, setting them down on the hot pavement next to his body. He was unresponsive but breathing so we went to work, stabilizing his spine and placing him on a backboard for transport to the hospital. While the ambulance crew prepared their stretcher, I continued my assessment of his injuries. He had minor abrasions to his scalp, which were still seeping blood, but overall, his small body appeared untouched. It wasn't until I checked his pupils that I became aware of the extent of his injuries.

Checking the equality, dilation, and reaction of the pupils is standard in assessing the level of consciousness of a patient. Certain conditions leave telltale signs within the pupils. Certain drugs will cause constriction, others dilation. The fixed and dilated pupils of the dead can be a haunting sight. But some of the most telling injuries read from the pupils are those involving the head. The eyes truly are windows to the soul. They are also windows to assessing brain function.

As I took a closer look at the boy, trying to determine the source of his unconsciousness, I reached to my belt to retrieve my penlight. These are the small flashlights carried in the field, used for such tasks as checking pupils, looking for foreign objects in various body orifices, and finding your way back to bed in a dark dorm. I checked the boy's right pupil, which was normal in diameter and sluggishly reactive. But when I checked the left, I was struck with an image that became fixed in my mind for days. The eye itself had begun to bulge and the pupil was grossly dilated and unresponsive. It seemed out of place on that serene face; it shone like some hideous anomaly, monstrous in nature. I checked it again, just to get a second look. I had never seen one eye appear so different from the other in an otherwise injury-free face. But this wasn't the first time pupils associated with a head injury had shocked me. One other patient sticks out in my mind.

I was working as a paramedic at Orlando Regional Medical Center, the city's Level I trauma center. The young black boy had been flown in via helicopter from a location outside the city limits. He had sustained massive head injuries after being struck by a car and was in full cardiac arrest by the time he arrived. Resuscitation efforts were unsuccessful and he was pronounced dead. It was my job to prepare the body for viewing, since the family had just arrived and been informed of his death.

The room was a mess. He lay on blood soaked sheets, with surgical tools strewn among bloodied tables. The wounds from his head had been intense and he had virtually bled out from the injuries, the majority of his blood ending up on the floor beneath him. The janitorial crews, who are specially trained in the cleanup of biohazardous materials like blood, urine, and human tissue, came in and efficiently scoured the floor. Now all that remained was his small form lying on the table, his blank eyes staring up at the overhead lights.

When the brain is severely injured, like any tissue it begins to swell. This swelling can cause a range of associated injuries, from temporary paralysis to permanent damage and death. Sometimes the swelling can be rapid and profound. Such was the case with the boy. Although he had expired, the swelling in his brain continued and within thirty minutes, the massive swelling had caused his eyes to bulge within their sockets. His pupils were rimmed in white, giving his face a look of intense fright. I knew this would be the image burned into his family's memory.

They entered quietly and approached the body, their hands protectively covering their mouths as their eyes took in his small form. I saw them staring at his face, unconvinced that this was their son who, hours before, had been running and playing in the street. I slipped out of the room and left them to their grief.

The eyes of the blond boy haunted me. For days I couldn't get his image out of my mind. I would lie in bed at night, re-creating the scene in my head. It always ended with his awkward stare. It took several days for me to remember that his eyes were blue. It was as if the color had escaped my notice until my mind had a chance to piece it back together. Two days later, I read his obituary in the paper. He was ten years old.

REGULARS

The thing I loved most about EMS was the ever-changing nature of each shift. I never knew what events would unfold from hour to hour. Every day was different; no two calls were ever the same. Most jobs seem mundane in comparison.

My short attention span was the result of my transient upbringing. I grew up a navy brat, moving every two or three years as my father progressed through the ranks. Even as a small child, I had little tolerance for regularity. No matter how content I was, after a year or so of being in one place, I would inform my father I was ready to move on. This trait carries over into most areas of my life, for I seem to have the attention span of a fruit fly.

EMS quenched my need for change. I loved not knowing what would transpire with each shift, never knowing when the tones would go off. We were always being summoned to some calamity, some situation needing resolution. There was great satisfaction in arriving on scene, mitigating an incident, and returning to service.

There were some aspects of the job that could be counted on for their regularity. Equipment checks, truck maintenance, and the paperwork associated with both, were stabilizers within shifts of uncertainty. There were also the regulars.

The term "regulars" was bestowed on anyone who frequently called 911. They generally called for the same complaint. The more creative individuals concocted new complaints with each incident. These were usually transients living on the streets who knew that a surefire way to a warm bed and hot food was not waiting in line at the local homeless shelter, but calling 911 and being transported to the hospital. There they could sleep on clean sheets and receive a bit of attention, small luxuries when you are penniless and without shelter.

We had many downtown regulars. Most were friendly and we dealt with them with familiarity and tolerance. Some were just plain scary. One individual, a heavy-set man in his fifties who had returned from Vietnam physically intact but mentally broken, would wander into local businesses, scaring the shit out of the clientele and forcing the owners to summon the police. The police would call us in and stand by as we tried to calm him, their hands cocked above their pepper spray.

The patient had a menacing look about him. His small gray eyes bored into you and he always looked on the verge of swinging. He frequently dropped hints about his latest unlawful act. On one occasion, he whispered to me how he had recently killed a man, describing the location of the dumpster where he had ditched the gun. I never knew whether to take these confessions seriously. We handled him with caution and usually turned him over to the officers for transport to the local psych ward. The last time I saw him, he was being put on a bus to Tampa, the ticket compliments of one of our investigators.

Most of our regulars were benign. They typically had chronic medical problems or were addicted to drugs or alcohol. They would call when it was cold, when it was raining, or when they were simply tired and hungry. We would chat with them a while and then direct them to the nearest shelter, sometimes coercing the police officers into giving them a ride. This minimized the likelihood of getting called back later that night.

One of our regulars was severely handicapped. He had been born with spina bifida, which left him significantly stunted, deformed, and confined to a wheelchair. He suffered from regular infections and we often found him at the local shelter, feverish and hungry. I can still remember the slightness of his weight as I lifted him from his chair, placing him carefully on the stretcher and padding his backside in an attempt to make him comfortable.

I also remember driving through downtown one evening and catching a glimpse of him on the sidewalk. He sat crumpled in his wheelchair, bent over and making slow progress down the sidewalk. I called out to him, asking him how he was doing. He replied back "I'm hungry!" My partner and I had just picked up hot meals from a local restaurant and were heading back to the station to enjoy a quick dinner. But his pitiful shape in that dilapidated chair overwhelmed me, so I had my partner circle the block. We pulled alongside him and I jumped from the truck, carrying the large meal of chicken and hot vegetables. As I placed it in his lap, his eyes lit up like a child being handed a brightly wrapped present. I waved and returned to the truck. Sometimes it's not how quickly you respond, the drugs you administer, or the lifesaving techniques you employ. Sometimes all it takes is a hot meal.

THE USUAL SPOTS

JUST AS EVERY TERRITORY HAS REGULAR PATIENTS, THERE ARE ALSO certain addresses that become regular spots for emergency calls. For Station 2, ours were the homeless shelter, which was conveniently located across the street, and the Lamar Hotel, a multistory, dilapidated hotel that provided grungy rooms for fifteen bucks a night. Ironically, they were located a block from each other. Someone on the downward slide into homelessness could simply gather his few belongings from the Lamar and proceed down the street to the shelter. There, his stained mattress was replaced by a green outline on the concrete, which delineated one's personal territory within the shelter.

The homeless shelter was a large block building with an open screened area where the men slept. There was an attached building that provided enclosed rooms for women and children. The women's shelter was stuffed with bunk beds, which were littered with shopping bags full of clothing and personal belongings. The women would greet us in various states of repose, sitting among the litter on the floor or lounging on their bunks, their legs hanging over the sides as they watched us work on patients.

We were usually called to the men's area, since they frequently took out their aggression on each other. Aside from the assaults, the building was a virtual breeding ground for infectious disease. A large proportion of the visitors suffered from tuberculosis, HIV, or both. A resounding chorus of rattling coughs could be heard throughout, and I often found myself holding my breath in a vain attempt to ward off the foul air.

The men were allowed inside late in the afternoon and hustled out each morning. They would begin to line up at the door around three o'clock so that they could claim the most desirable square, typically those closest to the windows. Once settled, they would inch their way through the food line for their one hot meal of the day. They would recline within their squares, talking to each other or themselves, until they somehow managed to doze off. It amazed me how anyone could sleep in such conditions, but I guess a square of concrete with a roof beats an open sidewalk any day.

There was an outdoor communal area, which consisted of a small dirt courtyard and several crumbling benches. The men would stand around and smoke, discussing their misfortune and blaming the current administration for their lousy lot in life. There was frequently liquor, which they would pass around, along with whatever infection they were currently battling. It was a scary place.

Since it was located just across the street from our station, we would often fantasize about building an elevated walkway so that those with medical complaints could simply walk over instead of repeatedly calling us out. The most infuriating were the calls in the middle of the night for some slight injury or ailment sustained earlier in the day. The patient would sober up enough to realize he had a cut that demanded immediate medical attention, albeit at 4:00 A.M. We would respond, bleary-eyed, and question him in disgusted tones before bandaging the wound and advising him not to call back. Sometimes it worked, sometimes it didn't. I once responded to the same person five times in one shift. By the fifth call, I was ready to kill.

It was always better to try to maintain a sense of humor when dealing with places like the shelter. I tried to empathize with the residents, but it was difficult, since many of the men were there by choice. For many it was a way of life that required no effort, no responsibility. They only had to withstand their dismal surroundings, but they didn't seem to mind. Many didn't want to hold down regular jobs and found the accommodations adequate.

Not all were there by choice. Many at the shelter were addicts. Many were psychiatric patients who had no insurance and so were deemed untreatable. Many were violent offenders released from prison, just waiting for an opportunity to exercise the very tactics that had landed them in jail in the first place. It was a rough and intriguing crowd.

The Lamar Hotel wasn't much better. In some ways it was decidedly worse. It had one main stairway that twisted and turned upwards, leading to floor after floor of filthy accommodations. These were small, stale rooms with single beds and dirty sheets. I don't know if the hotel restricted its clientele to men, but I rarely saw any women. The few women we treated were typically prostitutes who had been beaten while trying to make a hasty retreat or those who had overindulged in drugs or alcohol. The place was full of dirty, desperate men, many of them on drugs, most of them drunk. Violence was common, as were traumatic deaths, including beatings with pool sticks and hangings. We typically responded to the Lamar several times a shift. Each call evoked a sense of dread when the address was announced over the radio.

When we finally got word that the Lamar was to be torn down to make way for a brand-new office building, we were thrilled. So thrilled, in fact, that our department made arrangements to use it as a training facility where we could practice high-rise building tactics and forcible entry. It was strange to see the building free of drunks and addicts. The things they left behind, typically soiled clothing and large piles of shit, provided additional obstacles to our training, but we learned to look before we stepped and the structure proved to be an excellent training ground. It gave us great joy to tear open the doors and crash through the windows of a building that had been the source of so much aggravation. What once had been a middle-class hotel in the early 1900s had become a source of scorn for the emergency workers forced to frequent it. We were all too happy to see it go.

MISSING

One of our firefighters, John, was missing. Not in a fire, lost and disoriented by heat and smoke. Not stranded in a wildfire, cut off from rescue. He had gone fishing. He and his brother, JO, also a firefighter with the city, had taken a small boat out onto Tampa Bay to spend the day on the water.

Their afternoon had been uneventful, the success of their trip unknown. The details of the day were lost once John went missing. A storm had blown in with such speed they were unable to make it back to shore. As they struggled against the waves, their small boat capsized and they were thrown into the bay. JO fought against the churning waters and eventually made it to shore, but was unable to find John amid the dark swells. Word spread quickly.

John had come to the fire service late in life, having worked in various fields before finally attending the fire academy and obtaining his certification. He was tall, black, maintained the musculature of a young man, and spoke in quiet tones. He was intelligent, eager to learn, and would offer assistance at the slightest provocation. He had a warm smile and emulated kindness. It still amazes me that someone so strong could drown.

As soon as the news spread, our department mobilized and the Dive Team was assembled. Many came from home to gather equipment, ready their gear, and begin the long ride to the coast. Tampa firefighters were already on scene initiating the search, fueled by the anxiety that it was one of their own in the water.

As the sun set, there was still no sign of John. The search continued through the night. The divers would drag themselves from the water to sip hot coffee, eat a bit of food, and then return to the boats to comb the dark waters.

By morning everyone had accepted the fact that he had drowned. But the group refused to leave him behind. It was decided that efforts would continue until the body was recovered. The search went on.

I headed for the bay with several other firefighters, hoping to assist in some way since John and I had been stationed together when he was a rookie. I have a wonderful picture of us, filthy, sweaty, and smiling with satisfaction following a particularly intense fire one frosty winter night.

We arrived at the bay in early evening, and the dark skies were smeared with gray and blue from another afternoon storm. The wind was biting and we pulled our jackets tightly around our shoulders in an effort to ward off the cold. The divers continued searching the shoreline while small boats combed the bay, scanning its surface. Members within the command post studied tide charts and monitored the currents, trying to predict where the body might surface. The search went on for three days. Finally, on a beautifully clear, crisp morning, his body was spotted just off shore and pulled from the water.

Members of our Dive Team gathered as they brought him to shore, lifting John from the craft and carrying him to an awaiting ambulance. They moved like pallbearers, still dressed in their dive suits, their faces wet and salty. The groups eventually disassembled, silently gathering their equipment, shaking hands, and saying good-bye.

Although John didn't die in the line of duty, his funeral resembled the grand event of one who had. Firefighters came from across Florida, having heard of the communal effort on the shores of the bay. His body was carried on the back of a fire truck as hundreds of emergency personnel stood by in polished shoes and shining brass. John's death stood as an example of the bonds within the firefighting community.

I still wonder what happened out on the water that day. I picture him struggling against the waves, determined to grab hold of the boat, yet unable to reach it. I imagine his strong body fighting against the cold waters and the look of resignation that must have settled on his face as he slipped beneath the surface. One of the haunting aspects of working in the field of emergency services for so long is the ability to imagine, in all its frightening detail, the moment of death.

THE PATIENT

WORKING ON PATIENTS IS ALWAYS CHALLENGING. I HAVE ALWAYS loved medicine and it was this love that led me to the field of EMS. Some of the calls we run are painful; many of them are tragic. But when one of your own becomes the patient, it can be downright hilarious.

Mark had felt fine all afternoon. We had spent a quiet afternoon killing time, talking and laughing as we sat around the picnic table out back where we spent many hours bullshitting the time away, looking out onto the pleasant view of the littered vacant lot next door where the transients frequently urinated. It was a lovely afternoon.

But following our usual hearty dinner, Mark began to notice a subtle rumbling in his abdominal region. Thinking nothing of it, he excused himself several times in an attempt to relieve his body of whatever was about to wreak havoc on his system. It didn't work. In no time at all he was running for the bathroom, accompanied by the sounds of our laughter.

Firefighters are ruthless when it comes to humor at each other's expense. As we gathered upstairs to go to bed, we tried to take Mark's mind off of his troubles by making frequent jokes about his condition. The sounds of his retching blended with the sounds of his bowels exploding and he was soon miserable enough to pull his gear from the truck and retire for the evening. Knowing he would never make it home without ruining the interior of his car, he decided it would be best to camp out at the station and wait for things to improve. This was a great idea for him, not so great for me.

I had been assigned the less-than-desirable bunk just outside the bathroom door as a rookie at Station 2. The bathroom was a large room with showers at one end and sinks, toilets, and urinals at the other. Thankfully, my bed was near the shower end of the room. I hoped the distance would serve as a buffer against the racket of Mark's illness, but to no avail. All night I was subjected to the grotesque sounds of his vomiting and diarrhea. He would just make it to bed and be hit by another bout, which would force him to scurry back to the bathroom, dressed only in his underwear. (To add to the horror, he wore tighty-whities, which in my opinion should be outlawed for anyone above the age of twelve.)

Once relieved, he would creep back to bed, only to be forced into flight a few minutes later. After a while, the distance between his bed and the bathroom became too great, so he settled into the bed next to mine. As he lay nearby, groaning in between sprints to the bathroom, I took pity on him and spent the remainder of the night bringing him cool cloths for his forehead and water to keep him hydrated. In the morning, he quietly thanked me as he slowly made his way out of the station and home to bed.

THE INTRUDER

Someone had been tampering with our equipment. The incidents were irregular, but were occurring with greater frequency. We would find hoses uncoupled, regulators disconnected from air bottles, and other indications that someone had come into the station and handled our equipment. Perhaps it was supposed to be a joke. But running to the front door of a house fire and strapping on your mask only to find that your regulator has been disconnected is never funny. As the incidences mounted, so did our concern.

So our investigative division decided to mount a surveillance camera in the bay in order to catch the perpetrator in the act. This "secret" camera was quickly discovered by our personnel. We never thought it would be used to catch one of our own.

It was late at night on the tail end of another busy shift and the engine and rescue had been responding to a steady flow of calls. One of the men on the ladder truck, Dan, would regularly stay up late into the night, listening to calls going out around the city. He was constantly waiting for "the big one," the ultimate building fire; he was completely eaten up by the job. It was during his watchfulness that he caught a fleeting glance of someone running from the interior of the station as the rest of us responded to a call late that night.

He had followed us out into the bay as our trucks pulled out of the station in order to shut the doors behind us. As he walked out, he noticed someone slipping out of one of the bay doors and quickly heading south down the sidewalk and away from the station. He ran outside, trying to catch a glimpse of him, but the man, accompanied by a second individual, picked up his pace and they disappeared into the neighborhood.

When we returned from the call, Dan was anxiously pacing within the bay, waiting to fill us in on the latest drama. We huddled in the kitchen, wondering what we should do about the incident. Dan had surveyed the bay and adjoining rooms and could find nothing out of place. We looked over our trucks for any sign of tampering, but came up with nothing. Perhaps it was merely transients from the neighborhood looking for a dry place to sleep. Then we remembered the camera.

Firefighters are extremely clever. When faced with a problem, they strategize. It only took about five minutes for the guys to track down the main component of the camera, turn it off, and remove the tape. We inserted it into the VCR and began our investigation. Because it was a slow-recording tape, the images were captured in high speed. We had to watch it several times before we found the exact spot where a dark blur was shown exiting the bay. After several attempts, we were able to stop the tape just as the figure emerged. We slowed the tape and were amazed at what we saw.

The individual turned out to be one of our firefighters, Earl, who worked at a station across town on another shift. We tried to image what he would be doing in our station in the middle of the night. Surely he couldn't be the one tampering with our equipment. There had to be some other explanation for his presence. As we watched the tape, it soon became clear.

Earl hadn't been in the station to tamper with equipment. He hadn't been in the station alone. He was there to use our workout room, located on the other side of the bay, for a late-night rendezvous with one of his girlfriends. We watched as the two of them slipped out the bay, the majority of their clothing in hand, before fleeing down the sidewalk. Apparently our call had interrupted their date; we found one of the workout mats still streaked with sweat from their meeting, so we shot him an email asking him to please clean up after himself if he was going to use our station as a hotel room. Poor Earl never lived it down.

The source of the equipment tampering was never discovered.

LEARNING TO DRIVE

The earliest forms of fire engines were not engines at all; they were hand-drawn carts used to transport water to fires. Once the weight of the equipment became too heavy to be drawn by hand, horses were implemented. Early fire trucks relied on hand pumps to force water through the hoses, but were later replaced by coal-burning boilers. Today, we have diesel-powered engines capable of pumping thousands of gallons of water per minute through large-diameter hoses and specialized nozzles.

After several years on the job, I began the nerve-wracking process of preparing for my first promotional exam: engineer. The engineer's primary responsibility is driving the truck and supplying water to crews fighting the fires. They must know every inch of their rig and be able to manage multiple hose lines flowing various amounts of water all at one time. The promotional exam is intensive. Personnel are tested in three areas for competency. The first is driving. The driving course is a timed exercise and consists of a complex setup of lines and cones through which the candidate must maneuver the engine. The trick is to not cross the lines or squash any cones; each infraction deducts points from the overall score.

The second portion of the exam is a written test on fire tactics and standard operating procedures. Since engineers are permitted to "ride out of grade" in place of lieutenants, they must be able to assume responsibility for the truck and crew and supervise on-scene activities. Knowledge of SOPs is critical. This portion tests the candidate's ability to apply tactical knowledge to various types of emergencies.

The final portion of the exam is a practical exercise in hydraulics, which takes place on the training ground. The engineer is responsible for controlling the flow of water on a fire scene and must therefore have the ability to supply the needs of firefighting crews without running out of water. They must balance the amount of water exiting the truck against the amount coming in from hydrants. At a major event, with multiple lines flowing, it can overwhelm even the most cautious tactician.

The hydraulics practical consists of a large-scale scenario that will eventually force candidates to exceed the capabilities of their equipment. The key for the participant is to handle the event as it unfolds, secure the water supply so that he or she can flow multiple lines, and notify "command" when maximum output has been reached. The candidate can then request additional support. The assessors are officers from outside departments who are well versed in hydraulics, have extensive knowledge of fire-ground tactics, and are blessed with the ability to scare the shit out of candidates.

My promotional exam went smoothly. I completed the driving course in good time and without a single cone fatality. The written exam was a piece of cake, since I have always loved the beautiful coordination of fire-ground tactics and had crammed for months in preparation. The hydraulics portion turned out to be every bit the stressful event I had anticipated.

I pulled the engine up to the base of the tower, which would serve as the fire "scene." I set the parking brake, put the truck in pump, and then put it in gear so that it could achieve the necessary rpm's to run the pump.

I stepped out of the truck, ready for action. My assessor gave me my first assignment, which was to pull a 1¾" line from the truck. The 1¾" line is the standard size hand line for attacking most fires. Fire hoses are designated by their interior diameter, which determines their output. I pulled the line and flaked it out, removing any kinks in the hose that would prevent the steady flow of water. Once the line was on the ground, the assessor ordered me to pull a second line. This is where they hope to trip you up.

It's a law of fire-ground tactics that you *never* supply a second line without first establishing a water supply. This is done by hooking up a large-diameter intake hose from the engine to a nearby fire hydrant, opening the hydrant, and providing a steady inflow of water to your truck. In the stress of testing, the candidate can easily forget this rule, and many have failed by charging their second line without first securing the supply. I didn't fall for it. I hooked into the nearby hydrant, had water flowing into my truck, and then pulled the second line and charged it. Then things really began to move.

Before I knew it, my assessor was barking orders, yelling that the (imaginary) crews inside the fire needed more water. This tactic is meant to confuse candidates enough that they forget how many hoses they've established and how much water is flowing. The assessor typically sits back at this point, a big grin on his face as the candidate overextends the truck's capabilities and "cavitates" the pump. Cavitation occurs when the water supply cannot keep up with demand. Air enters the pump and the result is a blood-curdling grinding that sounds like a dryer full of rocks. It's a humiliating experience for the pump operator; the assessors live for cavitation.

Luckily, I somehow kept up with his furious barking and was able to juggle the supply and demand of the scenario without destroying the pump. I eventually reached the point where I was unable to supply more water and informed him that additional trucks would be needed to continue operation. This was just what he was looking for. With an approving smile, he ended my scenario and I walked away on weak knees, thrilled to be finished. I achieved an overall score that placed me number four on the promotional list out of almost thirty candidates. It was a great feeling of accomplishment and would set the stage for my future promotional exams.

DRIVING

IF YOU'VE EVER THOUGHT DRIVING IN HEAVY TRAFFIC IS STRESSFUL, you should try maneuvering a truck that's as big as a school bus, filled with 500 gallons of water, carrying specialized equipment and a pumped up crew, with sirens screaming and air horns blasting. Aside from the fact that the trucks cost around half a million dollars and the department is counting on your proficiency to avoid plowing into a building or taking out a group of pedestrians, driving a fire truck is one of the most exhilarating experiences on earth.

I was an engineer for two blissful years before being promoted to lieutenant. Racing through downtown Orlando on the way to a fire or medical call was the most fun I ever had on the job. I loved the fact that I was responsible for the safety of my crew, that they also depended on me to provide them water during a fire. I also loved all the gadgets.

A fire truck, or "engine" as it is commonly called, is extremely complex. It serves as a portable water supply with built-in pumps that enable the operator to elevate the pressure in the hoses so that an adequate flow can be maintained. Without the proper pressure, the water is unable to form an adequate stream. With too much pressure, the firefighters on the end of the hose line become airborne. One of the training exercises performed during the fire academy is called the "wild line," which teaches students how to gain control of a loose line. The instructors remove the nozzle from the end of a hand line, jack up the pressure on the truck, and then watch as the cadets frantically work their way down the line to gain control. The students inch their way along, squirming on their bellies as if they were wrestling an anaconda, until they reach the end of the line and pin it to the ground. The end result is always a muddy, soaked mess, but provides a nice break from the sweltering heat of the training field.

The pump panel of the engine consists of numerous levers that open and close the hose lines and a throttle that controls the rpm's to the pump. Each line has a corresponding gauge on the panel, indicating the pressure within the hose. The engineer controls the pressure to each line through the careful adjustment of levers. A series of stacked lights indicate the level of water in the tank. Each light that blinks out causes an automatic elevation in the operator's blood pressure, as he or she stands there fretting over how much water is left and how soon a supply line will arrive.

Although fire-ground operations are complex and thrilling, nothing equals the excitement of responding to calls. The massiveness of the truck accompanied by the wail of sirens makes the blood rise to your cheeks and your heart race. The trucks are equipped with a wind-up siren controlled by a floor pedal on the passenger side of the truck. The lieutenant controls this siren and can wind it up to a deafening scream. My heart rate still jumps when I hear a siren's wail. It is familiar music.

Driving an engine would be sheer pleasure were it not for one factor: other drivers. They can make the job of an engineer pure hell. I have learned over the years that most people regard their rearview mirror as nothing more than a means of applying lipstick or checking for boogers. They forget that it is a necessary component of safe driving and that scanning mirrors is critical. If more people remembered this, there would be far fewer instances of emergency vehicles roaring up behind unsuspecting drivers. Whenever this happens, the driver's typical response is to slam on their brakes, which makes for pure excitement for all involved.

Stopping a large truck on a dime goes against all laws of physics. Aside from its mass, the engines are carrying hundreds of gallons of water. Fortunately, fire trucks are fitted with "baffles," which prevent the water from sloshing about and causing dramatic shifts in weight. I remember countless instances where I would blare my sirens as I approached a vehicle, only for the driver not to notice us until we could see the whites of his eyes, and this only because his eyes had become the size of saucers by the time he caught us in the rearview mirror. Instead of pulling over to the right, as we are all taught in driver's ed, these drivers' immediate instinct was to slam both feet onto the brake pedal. Once they had their vehicle down to a slow crawl and my crew members had peeled themselves from the windshield, the scared driver would carefully pull to the side and watch in annoyance as we passed, many times saluting us with a middle finger.

But for all the annoyance and the close brushes with death, driving an engine is a tremendous thrill and I wouldn't trade the experiences I had behind the wheel for anything.

IN CHARGE

I WAS THE THIRD FEMALE IN THE HISTORY OF THE DEPARTMENT TO be promoted to the rank of lieutenant. It wasn't an easy process. The fire service is a testosterone-driven field where men are men and women are tolerated. When you think of a firefighter, you typically picture a buff, handsome male gallantly hanging from a ladder, single-handedly rescuing a family of five while controlling the inferno that has consumed their home. You typically don't think of a girl.

The first documented female firefighter was a slave belonging to a member of the Oceanus Engine Company Number 11 in New York City in the early 1800s. Making a reputation for herself as a hard worker, Molly Williams took her place among the men, distinguishing herself during the blizzard of 1818 by assisting crews pulling a pumper through the snow. Throughout the 1800s there are documented cases of women participating in firefighting, which typically led to honorary membership within their respective departments. The earliest professional female firefighters in America date to 1974. Our entry into the profession was still in its infancy when I was hired with OFD in 1988.

There were many obstacles to overcome in achieving the rank of lieutenant. The first was to obtain the necessary education, which was never a problem for me since I lived and breathed school. I had completed my officer's courses while still a firefighter, so I was more than prepared to take the next step—passing the lieutenant's promotional exam.

The exams are highly competitive and complex. The competition arises from the simple fact that males are involved. The complexity arises from the numerous areas in which the candidate is tested. These include fire tactics, administration, and standard operating procedures.

The first stage is a written exam that includes various aspects of the job, such as daily maintenance of crews and equipment, fire-ground operations, and policies and procedures. The next stage is the tactics exam. Here, the candidate is presented with fire and medical scenarios in order to gauge decision-making abilities and knowledge of standard operating procedures. It's a nerve-wracking experience. The scenarios are developed by departmental officers and consist of the most hair-raising incidents they can conjure. They typically involve phenomenal explosions, swirling clouds of hazardous materials, high-rise fires with victims dangling from windows, or some other godforsaken scene that is formulated within the depths of their devious minds. To make matters worse, there is always some unexpected development, such as massive equipment failures or the loss of your entire crew. Each scenario is timed, so the candidate must formulate a plan quickly and execute it before the clock runs out. This is meant to simulate the gut-wrenching pace of most emergency scenes. It's quite effective.

The final stage of the process is the administrative exam. This includes exercises in time management, prioritization, dealing with the public, and instructing other firefighters. Time management and prioritization are tested by dumping an overloaded "in basket" on the candidate, starting the clock, and having him or her wade through the piles of memos, events, and scheduling conflicts as quickly as possible. It is guaranteed to give the candidate a terminal ulcer.

Dealing with the public is tested by confronting an enraged civilian complaining that the fire department recently burned down his house, killing his dog and trampling his flowerbed in the process. Your job is to calm him down, deal with his issues, then send him happily on his way, all the while representing your department in the most professional light possible.

The final section tests the candidate's ability to assemble information in a logical manner and relay that information to a small class. The "class" consists of role players, typically personnel from the police department to ensure sarcasm and belligerence. As the candidate nervously proceeds through the lecture, the participants begin to heckle and cajole the instructor. They fight among themselves and act like spoiled children. It is the candidate's job to control the obnoxious students and complete the class without killing anyone. It's quite challenging.

I have been blessed with the ability to multitask. The exercises were fun for me. Being an anal-retentive individual and loving the juggling act of administrative work, I excelled and walked away with an overall score that put me in the top six on the promotional list. But my greatest challenges lay before me: commanding a crew on real emergency scenes.

My promotion was accompanied with the usual fanfare. I had to buy my entire station steaks and the firefighters subsequently doused me with a giant water gun following dinner. The latter was merely to show their love and affection, since acts of physical and emotional abuse are considered signs of endearment among firefighters.

My first assignment as lieutenant was on Engine 1. Station 1 housed two engine companies, a ladder truck, a heavy rescue, a district and division chief, as well as the department's special teams. It was a daunting task. I was thrust among highly trained individuals as I tried to fit in to a position of authority, all the while trying to conceal my anxiety over being in charge. They didn't make it easy. I had a great crew to work with, but there were several crew members at the station who seemed to resent the fact that a female had achieved rank before them. These individuals would challenge my authority, question my decisions on scenes, and basically flaunt their lack of respect.

It didn't deter me. I stood up to their challenges, never relinquishing authority and standing firmly behind my decisions. As time passed and I proved myself on emergency scenes, they eventually accepted my rank and moved on to other forms of entertainment. I settled into my new position, eventually growing comfortable with my authority but never forgetting the fact that they were watching and waiting for me to screw up. Being a female in a male-dominated field is like living in a fishbowl. You quickly learn to swim.

MEALTIME

One of the greatest bonding experiences among firefighters has nothing to do with emergency calls. It's not the rescue of civilians or the challenge of a fully involved house fire. It's dinner.

Most fire stations share at least one daily meal together, typically dinner. Dinner is a vital part of any shift. The planning begins early in the morning, when everyone is still settling in to the day's routine. At OFD, each station began the shift with a "morning meeting." During these meetings, the lieutenants advise the crews on the day's activities, such as building inspections, training, or special details. But the activity that takes priority over all is the planning of dinner.

There are typically several regular cooks at each station. These individuals are gifted with the ability to fix hot food in quantities large enough to feed an army, all the while being able to withstand the barrage of criticism that typically follows a fire department meal. The crews are not always cruel. They might even compliment the chef on his ability to grill ten pounds of steak in between running emergency calls. But God help the individual who messes up. Should the bread burn or the vegetables come out mushy, the cook has to endure a litany of complaints and verbal abuse. On rare occasions, the offending food ends up as projectiles as the crews compete to see who can hit the trashcans with greatest accuracy.

I cooked on occasion, but was not one of the regulars. It only took me a few attempts to prove my deficiency in the kitchen. First, I was not used to cooking for the masses. I generally cooked only for myself at home, so the prospect of having to feed a mass of hungry firefighters was daunting. There were several occasions when I came up short and the guys would harass me about the "dainty" portions. Next was my tendency to fix "light and healthy" cuisine. This never settled well with the crews. Although they appreciated a wholesome meal, they generally preferred quantity to quality, and my dinners usually left them rooting around in the kitchen an hour later for something more to eat.

But there were some fabulous cooks at the fire station. Each individual had his own specialty. Some were great with the grill. Those who were brought up in ethnic households would prepare great regional dishes that broke up the monotony of the typical American fair. Homemade pizzas loaded with vegetables and meats, steaming cauldrons of thick spaghetti, steaks the size of dinner plates, and roasts the size of small children were some of the specialties of the house. And nothing ended the day like a great meal accompanied by the animated conversations of the crews.

TRAINING

Training is an integral part of the fire service. Major incidents don't occur with enough regularity to keep skills sharp, so training sessions are vital necessities on any department. These sessions usually bring together several "companies." A company consists of a crew, whether it is assigned to an engine, a ladder truck, or a rescue truck. OFD standard operating procedures combine companies within rigid guidelines to accomplish tasks during emergency incidents. These combinations vary, depending on the type of incident.

The primary tasks at any fire scene include the attack of the fire (performed by the engine company), the removal of victims and ventilation of the building (performed by the truck and rescue company), and the treatment of victims (again, the rescue company). But the tactics depend on the scenario. Typical house fires involve two engine companies, a truck company, a rescue company, and a district chief to oversee the operation. High-rise incidents in buildings over three stories tall require more companies and greater coordination, since they are far more complex than residential house fires. Apartment fires utilize a combination of residential and high-rise tactics, since crews are dealing with multiple living spaces within multiple stories.

It's this complexity that makes fire tactics so intriguing. Each incident must be dealt with expediently and safely, and multiple tasks must be accomplished simultaneously and in rapid succession. Any time lost on the fire ground can mean the loss of life or property. This is where training comes in.

The goal of training is to hone skills so that they become automatic. Whether it's deploying hose lines, setting up for extrication of an entrapped victim, or evacuating casualties, each scenario must be practiced so that mistakes will be made on the training ground and not during an actual incident.

Training is also dictated by the department's Insurance Services Office (ISO) rating. The more training hours performed, the higher the rating for the department. Subsequently, the higher the rating, the more training hours required, so the two are interconnected. Needless to say, the amount of whining by the crew was directly proportional to the number of training sessions. During the more active training months, the griping would resonate throughout the city.

You would think firefighters would enjoy getting together to pull out their equipment and play with it a while. But Florida is known for one thing: eternal sunshine. This is great if you're a tourist coming down to tan your pasty-white northern skin. But if you're a firefighter, the heat can be intolerable. The weight of a full set of fire gear typically exceeds sixty pounds. It includes insulating pants and coat, boots, a helmet, as well as an air pack and facemask. This getup is great in a fire when you must be protected from the extreme heat of a flashover, but is can be pure hell in the Florida sun. The same gear that insulates you from the heat of a fire can act like the tinfoil surrounding a baked potato. You sweat like there's no tomorrow. Thus the dread of summer training. The last thing we wanted to do was don our heavy gear and prance around in the blazing summer heat. The sun would strike our black helmets like pounding fists, turning our brains to warm oatmeal and making concentration difficult. Following training, we would return to the station exhausted and dehydrated from baking in the sun.

Not all of the training was performed on the training ground. Sometimes training came in the form of videos we would watch at the station. We would gather in the cool of the TV room, settle into the big recliners, dim the lights, start the video, and doze for a while. It was blissful. There was no better break from the heat and pace of the day. Most of the training officers had prior experience with training "nap" sessions, so they typically kept video training to a minimum.

Later on, when I accepted an assignment to the Training Division as the lieutenant over EMS, I had the opportunity to train new recruits. The recruit classes lasted for several months and consisted of young, eager rookies chosen from a large pool of applicants. They had no experience in the field and it was the Training Department's responsibility to certify them as firefighters and EMTs.

It was great. Most of them were enthusiastic and idealistic and they absorbed each morsel of information like it was gospel. We introduced them to the warm and loving environment of the fire service by assigning them horrific nicknames, making fun of their clumsiness, and praising them on the rare occasions they did something right. They were good natured and tolerant, and it was always rewarding to attend their graduation as they were formally brought into the fold. I would see them, months later, as they were acclimating to their new assignments. They moved with newfound familiarity around the equipment, proudly wearing their clean, bright gear. Eventually they blended in with the veterans as they made their way through their careers, accumulating their own set of life experiences.

PRACTICAL JOKES

HUMOR IS THE LIFE'S BLOOD OF THE FIRE SERVICE. IT BRINGS CREWS together, it provides a release from stress and anxiety, and it passes the time during long, slow shifts. It's as if firefighters have a built-in mechanism that allows them to find humor in any situation. It's a necessity. The harsh reality confronted on the job gets to anyone after a while. Humor acts as a relief valve, letting the pressures of the job escape. It has a cleansing affect and allows each person a reprieve from the daily drama of EMS.

Firefighters find humor in each other. They prey on each other, digging beneath the surfaces of their macho exteriors to find anything resembling a weakness or insecurity. Once discovered, it is pounced on. Ridicule is a staple around the fire station and one quickly develops a thick skin. If not, you either crumble under the pressure or become alienated. It's sink or swim.

Rookies are immediately tested. They enter their new assignment timid and apprehensive and are immediately challenged in an attempt to single out anyone who exhibits a shred of sensitivity. Sensitivity is a killer. You must either refuse to let the harassment get to you or develop the skills of a seasoned actor. To reveal frustration or contempt is to open the door to a career of abuse. You have to roll with the punches.

Like all rookies, I was tested during my first months. In my case, it took a bit longer for the harassment to begin. Being a female, they were a bit more cautious, discerning what they thought they could get away with, making sure I wouldn't scream sexual harassment. Once they saw that I could take whatever they doled out and could dish it out in equal measure, the game was on.

The first incident happened late one night. I had gone to bed with the hopes of catching a few hours sleep, when I was called to the phone. I stumbled through the dark dorm, picking up the phone and wondering who could possibly be calling so late. It was no one. They had coated the receiver with shaving cream and called me from another line, just so I could smear the side of my head and be forced to drag myself into the bathroom to clean up. I took it in stride as remnants of the foam bubbled in my ear throughout the night.

The incidents that followed were as benign if not as annoying. I quickly learned that if you left your uniform shirt lying around the station, they would soak it in water and place it in the freezer. They presented me with my frozen shirt in a formal ceremony involving the entire station. I kept close tabs on my shirt from then on. They rigged laughing boxes under the toilet seat so that when I sat down, I had to relieve myself to the accompaniment of giggles. They lined my helmet with tinfoil smeared with motor oil so that when I donned my helmet, it resulted in hair that would put Elvis Presley to shame. It went on and on. I never let them see my annoyance. I good-naturedly laughed as I cleaned up whatever had been the focus of their latest prank. But paybacks followed and I reveled in my revenge.

I was raised in a family that thrived on laughter. That was what drew me to the fire service. The humor around the station was welcoming and familiar. I knew immediately that the fire service was for me. So prior to my first assignment at OFD, I was well versed in the art of pranks. I honed my skills at the fire academy.

I was the only female in my academy class, but that didn't stop me from partaking in the harassment typical of daily life at the academy. I would scheme with the best of them, always looking for an opportunity to tease or play tricks on my fellow students. It was on a hot afternoon heading back from lunch that I came upon a dead black snake lying in the grass near the training tower: a perfect opportunity. I quickly grabbed the snake, concealing it behind me as I made my way back to the tower.

The fire academy, like the fire service, is a paramilitary organization. They teach you the fundamentals of rank and order and you are expected to conduct yourself appropriately. You address your superiors according to rank and follow orders without question; daily life resembles boot camp. Following breaks, we would line up in formation, standing beside our gear, which was carefully laid out and ready to don. We would stand at attention as our instructors laid out the afternoon's drills. We would then assemble our gear and report to our assigned exercise.

I knew the routine. I knew the instructors would be standing in a line in front of us, looking us over with mock disgust as they barked out training assignments. They would then stand back and frown as we scrambled among our gear, always moving too slowly to suit them. The trick to boot camp is to not draw attention to yourself. That's why I chose to coil the snake under a particularly serious classmate's helmet,. Most of my classmates had seen me hide the snake, so they stood back, trying to conceal their laughter. As the cadet reached down and snatched his helmet from the ground, he noticed the large black snake coiled beneath it, ready to pounce. He shrieked like a schoolgirl, tossing his helmet high into the air, scattering his gear on the concrete. The helmet crashed to the ground, accompanied by the boisterous laughter of the class. The instructors responded with feigned disgust, berating the student, who took it in stride, shaking his head in embarrassment, his face burning with shame. The instructors never suspected me.

Pranks at the fire station took many forms. One of our district chiefs made the mistake of leaving his boat parked behind one of the stations while he went on vacation. It only took about a day for the boat to be relocated to the side of the road, a bright red For Sale sign attached to it. It was listed at a bargain price with the chief's phone number in bold print. He received many calls.

One of our rookies was informed that, since he was low man on the totem pole, during an EMS class to practice spinal immobilization skills he would play the "victim" and be immobilized on a long backboard. Once strapped down and unable to move, the rookie was quickly deposited in the dumpster out back as his crewmates stood by, laughing and taking pictures.

Our station had a balcony that overlooked the front drive. It was tradition for each rookie to be lured outside at some point, only to have a bucket of water dumped on his head. I somehow escaped this particular prank.

Beds were constantly rigged to antagonize the occupant. IV setups were concealed in the ceiling so that they slowly dripped onto the individual as he slept. Beds were filled with powder so that when the person got up in the night to respond to a call, he was blanketed in white. And my favorite prank:. underwear would be placed on the outside of bunker pants, which are kept assembled over the boots for rapid donning. The pants are pushed down around the ankles of the boots, which concealed the underwear until the owner pulled up his pants to secure the suspenders. By then, the truck would be pulling away from the station. The unwitting victim had no choice but to jump on board sporting his undergarments on the outside of his gear. The truly demented pranksters would use women's underwear.

But humor was a binding force among crews. It was part of the institution, like responding to calls or training. It came with the territory. The smarter ones accepted it, adapted, and learned from their experiences. What went around always came around and the traditions continue to this day.

HOME

If you ask any firefighter, he'll tell you his second home is the fire station. This is not because firefighters eat, sleep, and spend a third of their lives there. It's because it truly is like home.

The fire station is unlike any other workplace. It's not just an office; it's not a desk or a cozy cubicle. It's a place you come to know like your house or apartment. Every dark corner, every dusty closet, every damp bathroom within a fire station is a place of familiarity. It becomes a safe haven from the cold of winter, the heat of summer, and the stress of calls.

Each station has its own feel. The larger stations that house numerous companies are places of bustling, nonstop activity. There is always something going on. Each crew has its own responsibilities concerning truck maintenance, station duties, and administrative tasks. When I was assigned to the larger stations, it was impossible to get away from the constant buzz of activity. If you wanted privacy, you were forced to hide out in one of the small, upstairs offices. Here, you could actually enjoy a private phone conversation or a few moments of solitude. But it eventually happened that someone else in search of peace and quiet would stumble in on you, forcing you to wrap up your business and head back downstairs to the crowded rooms below.

The kitchens were popular places to congregate. In the morning, oncoming crews would mill around, meeting with off-going crews, crowding around steaming pots of coffee. Lunchtime usually meant squabbling over juicy leftovers from the previous shift's meal. Everything was first come, first serve, so you had to be quick. But dinnertime was the best.

The cooks would be hustling around the kitchen, trying to pace the preparation of the meal so that it would all be ready at once. The rest of the guys would be hovering around like vultures, sneaking tastes when the cooks weren't looking and pummeling them with verbal abuse because the meal wasn't ready yet. These were times of laughter, as we caught up on the day's events, sharing stories of earlier calls. The period before dinner was the time allotted for physical fitness, so many of the personnel usually wandered around in shorts and T-shirts.

Evenings following dinner were spent relaxing. We would assemble in back of the station, sprawled among old office chairs and picnic tables. Some would smoke. Others would sip coffee. The musicians would pull out their guitars, softly strumming as conversations waxed and waned. Slowly, one by one, we would filter off to bed, dragging our boots upstairs and settling into our bunks. We would speak in quiet tones so as not to wake those around us, and eventually each light would blink off.

It was a cozy feeling, sleeping in those large, cold dorms among fellow firefighters. We would settle in, hoping for a quiet night, hoping not to be startled awake by the tones. Sometimes, we would wake up in the morning, bleary eyed and amazed that we had slept through the night. Those were sweet mornings, waking up refreshed, gathering your belongings to prepare for shift change, meeting downstairs for coffee as the sun filtered into the kitchen. We would then say good-bye, heading off to our real homes.

I know I will never have another job like the fire department. I know no place will ever have the feel of a fire station, its rooms crowded with laughter and conversation. I will never feel the camaraderie of fire crews or the intensity of working beside people whom you trust with your life. These are the things that distinguish the fire service from all other occupations. It's what sets it apart from any other job and what made my time on the department like no other experience in my life. I look back over the years and can remember the feel of smoke in my throat, the weight of the gear on my back, and the intensity of the calls I ran. Nothing will ever replace my memories of the fire service. Nothing ever could.

PART THREE

COMMAND

LEARNING

Good timing requires effective communication.

—OFD SUPPORT ACTIVITIES

BY 1998, I WAS A NEW LIEUTENANT, I HAD NINE YEARS ON THE JOB, and I was restless. But restlessness had plagued me throughout my career. I always blamed my short attention span on my father. Growing up in a military family, moving every few years to a new location with new people, new places, and new cultures made repetition, for me, intolerable. Even in the fast-paced, ever-changing world of firefighting and EMS, the thought of spending twenty-five years doing the same job made me cringe. I combated this restlessness through education.

I didn't always enjoy school. High school had been one continuous party, interrupted only by weekends at the beach. I didn't consider myself particularly intelligent, and learning never seemed my forte, but I loved to read. My parents instilled in me the love of books and literature. My father entered the navy as a high school dropout and went on to complete a masters in theology from Northwestern University. He was an incredibly driven individual and spent his career traveling the world, reading great books, and loved working with people. I am him, incarnate.

Following high school, I lacked direction. I wasn't sure what I wanted to do, but I knew that once I figured it out, I would need the fundamentals. So I attended a community college, completing an associate of arts degree. It was during that time that I discovered anthropology.

Living overseas made me extremely curious about the world and people around me. When I was six, we moved to the Philippine Islands, where we lived for three years. The people amazed me: their customs, their dress, their language. Our housekeeper, Mara, shared many aspects of her culture with us, preparing exotic food, showing us traditional sewing techniques, and sharing stories she learned growing up on the island. Our house was located near the base perimeter, a high fence separating the modern Quonset huts of military officers from the poverty-stricken civilian neighborhoods. On weekends, I would stand outside and listen to the squeal of pigs as they were butchered for feasts. The air would fill with the intoxicating smell of roasting pork, and music would filter through the fence line. In the evenings, we would stand outside and watch bats descend from their daytime hiding places, swarming like dark locusts against the pale blue of twilight. The Philippines were a place of mystery to me, and I can still picture the lavender-colored mountains stretching beyond the airfields. My experiences as a military brat taught me to savor new places, new people, and to embrace change as a challenge and a way of life.

When I had completed my associate's degree, I went on to the University of Central Florida, majoring in anthropology. Anthropology, the study of man, is a four-field discipline and includes cultural and biological anthropology, linguistics, and archaeology. Each of these subdisciplines provides a unique yet integrated perspective in studying past and contemporary cultures. Cultural anthropology examines all aspect of human culture, such as religion and social structure; physical anthropology includes all of the scientific aspects of studying humans, from primatology to human evolution; linguistics examines the development, origins, and spread of human languages; and archaeology is the study of man via material remains. I was especially interested in bioarchaeology, a subfield of physical anthropology, which focuses on the analysis of human skeletal remains from archaeological sites. The subfield addresses issues of health, diet, and pathology among past populations. I would later specialize in bioarchaeology as a graduate student at Florida State University following my departure from OFD.

It was while studying anthropology at UCF that I decided to switch gears and become a paramedic. I knew the road to anthropology required advanced degrees, which intrigued me but also made me chafe. I wanted out of school. I wanted to be independent, to find a career that I could enter quickly, and an education I could complete sooner than later. So I left the university and entered paramedic school.

As a paramedic, you have two educational options. You can complete the shorter, less-rigorous certification program in emergency medical services, or you can complete the degree, which includes additional prerequisites and coursework. I chose the degree path. I knew the additional coursework would come in handy, should I decide to go on to other areas of medicine. I completed an associate of science degree in EMS just as I was applying for OFD.

Once I was hired by OFD, I pursued a degree in fire science. The degree included coursework in fire tactics, hazardous materials emergencies, building construction, and administration. These courses also fulfilled the requirements for becoming a lieutenant, which I intended to pursue as soon as I had accumulated enough seniority. OFD requires a certain amount of time on the job before personnel can pursue rank. At the time of my employment, you were required to be on the job for three years before taking your first promotional exam for the rank of engineer. You must also have been certified as a "relief driver" for one year prior to the engineer exam. Relief drivers were qualified to act as engineers, driving the trucks and fulfilling all duties and responsibilities of an engineer yet without the official rank.

To become a lieutenant, you had to have been an engineer for at least two years. These requirements insured that personnel spent time "riding out of grade," which meant serving in the role so that you would be prepared for the rank by the time you obtained it. It also provided "training grounds" for up-and-coming officers. Someone on a fast track could join the department, take the engineer's exam after three years, and then take the lieutenant's exam after being an engineer for two years.

It was while pursuing my fire science degree that I decided to complete my bachelor's in anthropology. I returned to UCF and continued my coursework. But I also was thinking of a life beyond the fire department. Since medicine had always intrigued me, I considered pursing medical school. During the two years I spent at UCF studying anthropology, I continued coursework toward my fire science degree. During the summers I worked toward obtaining premed requirements, which included additional courses in biology, chemistry, and microbiology. It was during one of these summers that I decided to look into orthopedic surgery as a potential future occupation.

I loved the field of orthopedics. I was always fascinated by the human skeleton and had watched with amazement as the orthopedic surgeons worked on trauma patients in the emergency room. Their skills astounded me and their use of traditional tools, such as hammers and screwdrivers to mend broken bones and shattered limbs, made for some of the most exciting medicine I had ever seen. So I contacted the head of the residency program at the Orlando Regional Medical Center and asked if I could "shadow" some of the orthopedic residents. It was a fascinating month spent following residents from case to case, working alongside them in the emergency room, and observing their techniques in surgery. I was even allowed to "scrub" on one occasion and assist in the debridement of a burn patient by holding the limb while the surgeons worked. But after a year-and-a-half of full-time coursework in addition to working for OFD, I was burned out and wanted to focus on the fire department. So I put off medical school and continued to juggle coursework in both degrees, completing my BA in anthropology followed by the AS in fire science, all the while pursuing the rank of engineer and then lieutenant.

School gave me focus. It challenged me in ways the department didn't. I realized I loved learning and that when I applied myself, I could take on any amount of coursework with success. I achieved the rank of engineer and was promoted to lieutenant two years later. Once I had achieved the rank of lieutenant, I set my sights on becoming only the second female district chief in the department. I knew I would need additional education to manage the administrative responsibilities of the position, so back to school I went, completing a master's degree in public administration through Troy University. Troy had a satellite campus open to civilians on the nearby navy base. I completed the degree in just over a year, becoming one of only a handful in the department with a graduate degree.

In addition to formal education, I also wanted to improve my skills as a firefighter. I completed Rope Rescue I, an intensive course in high-angle rescue and emergency escape. This course is designed to teach firefighters the skills used in above-ground rescues, which include utilizing an array of complex ropes and knots, along with advanced skills in rappelling. Students are taught how to secure tools and equipment during elevated rescues, how to secure and lower patients from various heights, and how to perform emergency escapes from burning structures. The week is spent on hands and knees, scurrying through simulated fires and performing emergency escapes by rappelling head-first out of windows. By the end of the week, each of us was exhausted and bruised from shoulders to knees, but we left the course proficient in advanced techniques of elevated rescue. It was an exhilarating learning experience.

During this period, I also became a Hazardous Materials Medical Technician, a Critical Incident Stress Debrief provider, and a certified diver. My focus was education and I pursued any opportunity for knowledge and self-improvement. But it was during my first six months as a lieutenant that my perspective on firefighting was permanently altered. This event would change my view of firefighting and the risks that we face on a daily basis.

A HOLE IN THE FLOOR

Effective fire control requires that water be applied directly on the fire or directly into the fire area.

—OFD OFFENSIVE OPERATIONS

I BELIEVE EVERYONE IN EMS EVENTUALLY EXPERIENCES ONE CALL that changes them, that alters their perception of the job itself, making them question what they do for a living. Mine came about six months after being promoted to lieutenant. I was still assigned to Engine 1 at the time.

It was around 4:00 A.M. on a quiet weekday morning. I was awakened by the "hotline," the phone line that links our Dispatch Center to individual stations. I stumbled through the dark to pick up the flashing line. My engine was being sent to a smoke odor investigation. These calls typically involve cruising through the city, trying to sniff out an illegal burn or a homeless person's cooking fire. I gathered my crew and we loaded up. The call had come from one of the local emergency rooms. Hospital personnel had been standing outside, enjoying a quick smoke break, when they noticed a heavy concentration of smoke in the area. They called 911 and we responded.

We arrived in the area and I spoke to the ER staff, asking them how long they had smelled the smoke. They said the odor had been around for about forty-five minutes, but was becoming more intense. We headed west from the hospital into a small business district composed of large, converted Florida homes that now served as offices. The smoke was getting thicker.

We turned down a side street, our heads out the window, sniffing like bloodhounds, trying to determine the source of the fire. Different fires have different smells. You can typically determine the type of fire by the characteristic odors associated with the different materials involved. Wildfires have the rich, earthy smell of burning trees and ground litter. Car fires carry the acrid stench of burning polyester and metal. House fires are a combination of everything you can imagine: wood, plastics, clothing, and even human tissue. The sense of smell is a primary tool of a firefighter.

We slowed down as we approached a large, two-story Spanish-style house that had a For Lease sign on the front lawn. It was a vacant office building and it was definitely on fire.

Heavy smoke was puffing from the ground-floor rear windows. I called in a full alarm, advising Dispatch that we had a "working house fire." As the tones sounded over the radio, pulling crews from their sleep, we donned the rest of our gear and proceeded to the front door to make entry.

It started out as a textbook case: we would enter from the unburned side and make our way to the rear of the structure where we would force the fire out the back windows. Textbook cases always have a way of turning on you.

By the time we donned our gear and assembled our hose and equipment at the front door, we could hear the approaching wail of sirens as additional trucks came screaming through the city. As the trucks arrived, crews bailed off as the drivers slowed to position their rigs in front of the structure. My firefighter and I were joined at the front door by two crew members from Tower 1. We readied our hose line as they forced open the door. The front room was a small sunporch that opened, via double french doors, into a large main room. We crawled inside.

The smoke was extremely thick. We instantly lost sight of each other as the blackness enveloped us. Instantly I knew something was wrong. Heavy smoke is typically accompanied by an intense amount of heat, so much so that we are usually forced to crawl on hands and knees to avoid the heated gasses that rise with the smoke. But for some reason there was little heat. My stomach began to churn.

It's hard to describe the feeling of entering a dark, smoke-filled building you know is on fire. Your first instinct is to rush forward to locate the fire. But there are procedures that must be followed. OFD follows a "right-hand search" approach, in which you always maintain contact with the wall to your right so that in a pinch, you can turn around and retrace your way back out. As one crew advances the hose line, other crews ventilate windows and search for victims. Everything happens in concert.

So we entered the structure, stepping up into the main part of the house. That nagging feeling continued, and I quickly flipped through tactics in my mind, trying to settle on what type of fire would cause such intense smoke and so little heat. It was then that I noticed a faint, orange glow that appeared to be about twenty feet in front of us. I tapped my firefighter, yelling through my facemask for him to hit it with water. He opened the nozzle, releasing a quick burst of water then quickly closing the nozzle. This is known as a "thermal balance approach," where a quick burst of water is used to dampen down a fire by converting the heat to steam. The glow disappeared for a brief moment. We squinted through the smoke, trying to locate the fire when suddenly the room burst into massive shades of orange and red. I can still remember the fire against my facemask as the reflectors on my gear began to melt.

The flash pushed us backwards. I became separated from the others as I was forced to the left, they to the right. I began to back out toward the french doors, using my foot to try to locate the opening. Suddenly, my back was against a wall. Somehow the fire had forced me into a corner and away from the doorway. My brain was screaming for information. It was at this point that events began to come together.

The radio was alive with the high-pitched chatter typical of fire scenes, but through all the noise, I heard one voice call out "Basement fire, basement fire!" My first thought was "There are no basements in Florida!" Because of Florida's high water table, few structures are built with basements characteristic of older houses in northern states. In fact, I couldn't recall ever seeing a basement in a Florida home.

One of the crew members to my right began screaming for us to evacuate. His voice saved me. I used it as a beacon, crawling sideways toward the front door that had somehow shifted behind me when we positioned ourselves to open the nozzle. We scrambled out, dragging the line behind us as we exited the fully involved structure, collapsing in relief on the front lawn. I was never so happy to feel grass beneath my hands and knees. But I still couldn't appreciate how close we had come to catastrophe. We later retraced the events leading up to the fire.

Carpenters had been working in the basement the previous day. They had left their equipment behind, knowing they would resume construction the next morning. One of their soldering irons had set the room on fire, which burned for several hours before eventually snuffing itself out as it consumed the last bit of oxygen in the room. What it needed was a nice gust of fresh air, which was provided by a firefighter on the ladder truck when he located and entered the basement.

Upon arriving on scene, the firefighter from the ladder truck had done exactly what he was supposed to do: proceed around the structure to ventilate the windows near the seat of the fire. But as he made his way around the building, he noticed a small basement doorway. He made his way down the narrow steps, forcing the door and making entry. It was the opening of the door that ignited the contents of the room in a powerful flash. The fire shot up into the main room of the house via a huge burned-out area of the first floor, right as the four of us were entering the room. The fire mushroomed through the opening in the floor, filling the room in its entirety, flashing over us like an orange wave.

When the fire was finally under control and we were able to walk through what was left of the interior, we were amazed at how close we had come to stepping into the giant burned-out hole in the center of the main room. Had we taken a few steps forward, all four of us would have fallen in. The flashover would have enveloped us in flames. There would have been no escape.

We stared at that hole for a long time. My firefighter had just celebrated the birth of his first child. He was stunned into silence by how close he had come to leaving his daughter fatherless. When I returned home later that morning, I sat in the silence of my apartment, reflecting over the events of the morning. I had experienced close calls before. I had even experienced the loss of a fellow firefighter and friend who had been killed in a commercial structure when the ceiling fell in as he and his crew searched for the source. I had come to terms with the risks of the job. It was the potential waste of life that bothered me. The fact that the four of us could have been killed for the sake of an empty building was maddening. There were no victims needing rescue. Our deaths would not have been justified by heroic measures; they would have been for nothing.

This call changed my perspective of the job. It changed the way I looked at firefighting, the way I justified the risks firefighters take each day. In fire tactics, the concept of "risk versus gain" is a common theme and one that dictates decisions on the fire ground. When making tactical decisions, a commander must take into account the risk of personnel versus what can be gained by aggressive tactics. For example, in a structure with the potential for heavy loss of life, such as a nursing home, the risk of sending in personnel to fight a fire is justified by the gain of saving many lives. In the case of abandoned or dilapidated buildings, risking the lives of personnel in order to save such a structure is unjustified. Risk versus gain is fundamental to all fire-ground tactics.

It was perfectly reasonable to think about risking one's life for the sake of another. That aspect of the job instilled in me a sense of pride and duty, and to this day I feel firefighting is one of the most noble of professions. But the idea of losing one's life for the sake of an empty building rattled me, causing me weeks of introspection as to where I was in my career and where it was going. It was during this time that the chief of my department made me an offer that would change the direction of my career.

A NEW DIRECTION

When you cut a hole in a roof, cut a big hole.

—OFD SUPPORT ACTIVITIES

IT WAS LATE IN THE AFTERNOON WHEN THE CHIEF OF THE DEPARTment pulled up behind Station 1. I had escaped to the back patio area for a bit of quiet and to catch up on some reading. I was engrossed in a book about forensic anthropology when I looked up to see him approach.

He sat down and asked me how I liked being a lieutenant. I told him I was adjusting to the new rank, getting the hang of the additional paperwork involved. Lieutenants are responsible for maintaining records of all the training hours completed by their crew, as well as the day-to-day administrative paperwork of fire inspections and physical activity. These tasks are tracked and the hours totaled at the end of the month, all of which go toward maintaining the department's ISO rating. The ISO rating is based on the effectiveness of dispatching emergency calls, the number of emergency units in service, the level of training within a department, and the adequacy of a community's water supply. These ratings are then used by insurance companies to determine rates within a department's jurisdiction.

At the time, OFD maintained a rating of 2; they now maintain the prestigious rating of 1.

He then asked if I was happy on shift. I loved shift work. I loved the twenty-four-hour duty days and how each shift unfolded. The two days off in between were an added bonus and gave me ample time to go to school and study. By this time, I had just completed my master's degree in public administration. The chief was aware of this, of course. My reputation as a nerdy student was well known throughout the department and a constant source of teasing among the crews. I could usually be found with my nose in a book. The obscure topics I studied, such as bioarchaeology, genetics, and anthropology, typically produced puzzled expressions and the inevitable question, "What are you reading that for?" Since these topics had nothing to do with firefighting, most of the guys couldn't understand why I would spend hours reading about human skeletal analysis or evolutionary biology. But it was just that reason that I found them so interesting—not only because they were scientific, but because these subjects were far removed from my work as a firefighter. They were an escape for me and a means of expanding my knowledge base. They also symbolized a possible future direction, since I still hadn't accepted the idea of staying in the fire service for the full twenty-five years.

After our initial chitchat, he broadsided me with the question, "You want to go to Training?" He was offering me the position of training lieutenant, one of two administrative positions within the EMS Training Division. OFD's EMS Training Division operated like many training departments throughout the country; a district chief oversaw the department and a lieutenant was responsible for maintaining the paramedic and EMT licenses of all personnel, providing continuing education classes so that personnel obtained the required number of continuing education units (CEUs), and assisting with training new cadets—in other words, a tremendous amount of paper-pushing and an end to twenty-four-hour shift work. Training personnel worked a five-day workweek, something that was completely foreign to me, having been on shift for almost a decade.

Although surprised by his offer, it was something that had been playing in the back of my mind for some time. The reason I had completed a master's in public administration was to learn how to be a proper administrator. The role of a combat shift lieutenant had a fair amount of administrative responsibilities, but nothing compared to an actual administrative position within the department. I knew having experience in an administrative position would benefit my future. I would learn more about the inner workings of the department and put to use some of the skills I had developed during my degree program.

Also in the back of my mind were the recurring thoughts concerning the close call I had experienced. During the weeks following the call, I spent a lot of time thinking about my job as a firefighter. The feelings of restlessness had intensified, as if the call had increased my desire to move on to another career. It wasn't fear or an unwillingness to risk my life. It was more a feeling of wanting "something else." My restlessness had driven me to complete three degrees, yet I was still not satisfied. The close call had reminded me of the tenuousness and brevity of life. Having watched my mother die at the age of fifty-three, I felt a tremendous sense of urgency to take advantage of every opportunity and not waste time.

With each course I took and each book I read, I realized more and more that there were other things I could be doing with my life. I fantasized about leaving the department, entering a degree program, and just being a full-time student for a while. The thought of attending a university and focusing on a new area of study seemed blissful, and at times it took effort to remain focused on the department and my career within it.

So the thought of shifting gears within the department sounded like a nice change. Perhaps it would quell my restlessness by giving me a new area in which to work, a new suite of responsibilities to master, and an arena in which I could flex an intellectual muscle. I called the chief the next day and accepted the position. I was headed for the Training Division.

TRAINING DIVISION

We lose most often because of lack of support, not lack of water.

—OFD SUPPORT ACTIVITIES

I ENTERED TRAINING IN THE SPRING OF 1999. THE TRAINING DIVIsion was housed in a set of portable buildings located on the grounds of the fire academy. This provided close proximity to the training tower, a multistoried concrete-block building used for simulating fire and rescue scenarios. Also on site was the burn building, a bunker-like structure made from fire-resistant materials, built to withstand the extreme temperatures of training fires. The walls of the burn building were blackened from years of heavy fire, and walking through the structure was like walking through a burned-out cave: dark, damp, and smelling of soot.

It was a strange feeling returning to the fire academy as a training lieutenant. Looking across the grounds took me back to my months in the academy, running laps in full gear, sweating out countless push-ups, and working endless hose evolutions. My office was located in one of the portables. It was the first time I had ever had my own desk and work space. The offices at the stations are shared by all personnel, so the sense of ownership was a new thrill. But it was a minor thrill.

Immediately I longed for a return to shift. Reporting to an office every day smacked of the repetition I so loathed. But the new responsibilities were exciting, so I focused on the challenges and embraced my new position.

Working in administration brought me into contact with a very different circle. Shift lieutenants mainly interact with combat crews and their immediate superiors, the district chiefs. As a training lieutenant, I attended meetings of city and EMS officials, representing the department and speaking on its behalf. It was intimidating, but I came to appreciate interacting with people outside of the department. The various perspectives and concerns of other officials within EMS made me more aware of the complex interactions that make up a community's emergency medical system. In Orange County, all paramedics and EMTs are overseen by the county EMS office, which is run by a director, his or her staff, and a physician that serves as Medical Director for each agency. Paramedics and EMTs work under the Medical Director's license, and he or she serves as a reference point when personnel are faced with difficult situations in the field.

When I first became a paramedic, we were not permitted to stop resuscitative measures, such as cardio pulmonary resuscitation (CPR), without permission from a physician, either the Medical Director or an ER physician who was notified by radio. Now protocols provide greater flexibility for field personnel. If the patient meets certain criteria that are deemed "incompatible to life," such as decapitation, severe trauma, or rigor mortis, the paramedic has the ability to "call the code," or simply "call it," meaning stop all resuscitative efforts.

I learned a tremendous amount in my first few months in Training. Many of my days were spent running from meeting to meeting. My primary administrative duties were to oversee the paramedic and EMT licenses of all personnel. These licenses are regulated by a two-year cycle during which personnel must complete a required number of hours of continuing education units (CEUs). It was my responsibility to provide the necessary training and ensure that all licenses were kept up-to-date. Since paramedics and EMTs are required to stay current on the American Heart Association guidelines, which dictate the protocols for CPR and all advanced cardiac life support (ACLS) treatment, I completed instructor courses in CPR, ACLS, and Basic Trauma Life Support (BTLS). This enabled me to provide recertification courses for all OFD personnel. It also prepared me for another of my responsibilities as training lieutenant: training new recruits.

A new program had been implemented at OFD a few years before I was assigned to Training. The "cadet" program took untrained individuals off the street and certified them as firefighters and EMTs. The purpose for the cadet program was to improve representation of various minority groups within the department, primarily blacks, Hispanics, and women. I would train two cadet classes during my tenure in the Training Division.

I was responsible for the cadets' physical training (PT). Each morning began by lining up the recruits and taking them through a Navy SEAL's workout. The workout consisted of countless push-ups to build upper-body strength, stretching exercises to increase flexibility to avoid injury on the training ground, and, of course, endless running. The workouts were challenging and a great way to begin each day. It was also rewarding to watch the cadets improve over time. Many of them lost weight as the course progressed, becoming stronger and more self-assured.

By the fall, a second cadet program had begun and the two classes overlapped, one beginning at dawn, the second starting an hour-and-a-half later. During those months, I would arrive at the training ground before sunup and line up the first batch of bleary-eyed recruits. I would take them through their workout as the sun slowly rose and the second group of cadets arrived. When the first group had completed PT, I would dismiss them to the showers and begin working out the second group. That period put me in the best physical condition of my career. It was also incredibly rewarding helping shape the new members of our department.

Months later, when my first group had started shift work, I would see them on their rigs, blending in among the more seasoned firefighters, and it gave me a sense of pride knowing I had been a small part of their entry into the department. It also added another dimension to my leadership skills. Instructing fresh-faced cadets was quite different from dealing with the seasoned personnel on shift. It required a lot more patience, since these were kids who had no background in EMS or fire. They came to the program knowing nothing about the fire service other than they wanted to be a part of it. I remembered my academy training and the instructors who taught me the most. They were not the ones who yelled the loudest or browbeat the students the most frequently. They were the ones who patiently taught me how to be a professional. They led by example.

LEARNING TO LEAD

In all cases, the initiative and judgment of the Officer are of great importance.

—OFD COMMAND PROCEDURES

BY FAR THE MOST ADVANTAGEOUS ASPECT OF WORKING IN ADMINISTRATION was access to specialized training. Suddenly I was being sent to the most prestigious training conferences and programs in the country.

The National Fire Academy (NFA) was created in 1974 in conjunction with the U.S. Fire Administration. In 1971, President Nixon brought together a group of experts to address the growing problem of fire in the United States and to identify means of improving the training of firefighters. The group, known as the National Commission of Fire Prevention and Control, produced the landmark publication *America Burning,* which recommended the establishment of a national academy for firefighters. This academy would provide specialized training in arson investigation, incident command, and emergency scene management and would be free of charge. The government would cover the cost of the courses.

The NFA and the Emergency Management Institute (EMI) are located in the small town of Emmitsburg, Maryland, about twelve miles south of the famous battleground, Gettysburg. The town of Emmitsburg was founded in 1785 when Samuel Emmit deeded thirty-five acres of land to his son William. The NFA and the EMI are located on a beautiful campus that once housed Saint Joseph College, the first parochial school for girls in the United States. Founded in 1809 by Elizabeth Seton, the school closed in 1973 due to diminished enrollment and was purchased in 1979 by the U.S. government to house the Academy and Institute.

The campus, known collectively as the National Emergency Training Center, is located amid the rolling hills of northern Maryland. Flanked by fields of corn to the west and fragrant forests to the east, the historic red-brick buildings spread out atop a rich, green landscape. A few modern buildings serve as admissions and administration, and the dorms are immaculate structures that consist of private rooms and baths that house students during the two-week courses.

Courses provide intensive training in specialized areas of fire administration and emergency scene management. My first course was entitled Control of Fire Department Operations at Natural and Man-made Disasters. I arrived for my training late in the afternoon on a Sunday in late spring. I stood in line inside the admissions hall, the only female among a roomful of men from fire departments all over the country. After receiving our dorm keys and a map of the campus, we headed for our rooms to unpack and settle in.

I had heard about the NFA long before I applied for the course. Attending the Academy was a prestigious event in a fire officer's career, one that typically singled a person out as ambitious and upwardly mobile. There is a lengthy application process followed by months of waiting. I applied without mentioning it to anyone, worried I might not make it in on my first attempt. So to be roaming the vast campus was a thrill to me. I felt my career was on track and I was doing everything possible to hone my skills in incident command and emergency scene management.

The course involved classroom lecture and simulated emergency incident management. There were about thirty students in the class, most of them officers from departments of various sizes from around the country. The material was fast-paced and we were thrown into command scenarios almost immediately. During these scenarios, we would role-play various positions within the command structure, each responsible for certain aspects of scene management.

Emergency scene management involves a single incident commander overseeing various "sectors" within the command structure. These sectors can include medical, fire, and extrication, each overseen by an officer responsible for the activities within the sector. For example, the medical sector would oversee the treatment, "packaging," and transportation of patients at an emergency scene. Each sector reports to the incident commander. This ensures fluidity of scene management and reduces the chance of any one commander becoming overwhelmed.

Each student got the opportunity to act in various sector roles and the scenarios changed daily. The scenarios included high-rise fires, large hazardous materials spills, natural disasters, and mass casualty incidents. The final day of class consisted of a "major incident" conjured up within the satanic minds of our instructors. Each student was assigned a position within the command structure and we all worked in concert to mitigate the event.

To be on that beautiful campus, with the singular responsibility of attending class each day and studying each night, was what I had longed for. In addition to the coursework, being able to discuss tactics with members of departments from different parts of the country was educational and enlightening. The students represented departments from varying backgrounds, some urban, some very rural. Each department faced its own set of challenges. For some, it was limited manpower and equipment; for others, it was the environment. The departments ranged from Puerto Rico to Alaska. The social interaction at the academy was as enriching as the classroom.

My year in the Training Division provided numerous educational opportunities. I attended the NFA twice, the second time completing the course Emergency Medical Services Special Operations. At the Emergency Management Institute I completed IEMC/All Hazards Preparedness and Response, a course that brought together community-wide representatives to learn how to handle large-scale emergencies. At the University of

Maryland Fire and Rescue Institute I completed the National Fire Service Staff and Command Course. I also attended local training, including Terrorism Operational Planning in Orlando and Command School '99 in Daytona, Florida.

These courses, in addition to my AS in fire science and my master's in public administration, taught me how to approach emergency incidents in a thoughtful, methodical manner. It taught me how to manage resources, anticipate the needs of command, and to keep my cool when all hell is breaking loose around me. As in my fire science courses, the national curriculum reinforced the concept of risk versus gain. Over many decades of research, it was becoming apparent that firefighters had to improve the way they approached fire, replacing the "rush in" mentality with one that was more contemplative and one that weighed the potential gains versus the level of risk to personnel.

At OFD, this change in tactics was not immediately embraced. The traditional mentality of the department meant a commitment to aggressive, interior attacks: the red meat of firefighting. In most cases, these aggressive attacks were highly productive, locating victims expediently, bringing fires under control quickly, and minimizing property damage. But I had been on the department long enough to witness the overzealous interior attacks that put personnel at risk for the sake of structures that were either cleared of victims or already significantly destroyed.

Much of this was related to the mentality inherent to firefighting. The teasing and horseplay characteristic of the fire department environment tends to morph into a form of peer pressure when it comes to job performance. Those seen as cautious or solicitous tend to be regarded as outside the norm of traditional, aggressive firefighting. Many young firefighters who lack education, experience, or both, tend to develop tunnel vision when it comes to attacking fire. They disregard the scene as a whole, focusing only on getting "water on the fire." The primary objective to good tactical training is learning to take in the entire scene, to foresee events before they occur, especially those that endanger crews and hamper the objectives of scene management.

The year I spent in the Training Division and the tactical training I received at the NFA, EMI, and command conferences across the country instilled in me the essential objective of weighing risk versus gain at emergency incidents. These lessons, in addition to ten years on the job and the recent close call I experienced at the basement fire, imparted in me the requisite restraint a tactical commander should possess when sending personnel into hazardous situations. Ironically, it was this approach to tactics, acquired through training sponsored and encouraged by OFD, that would lead me to confront the reckless tactics I witnessed while fighting what would be the last fire of my career.

A FORK IN THE ROAD

If fire is working inside a concealed space,
get ahead of it, open up, and cut it off.

—OFD SUPPORT ACTIVITIES

As my first months in Training wore on, I settled into the position, enjoying the additional training and responsibilities. But regardless of these new experiences, one thought kept creeping into my mind: leaving. I still grappled with the restlessness that had followed me throughout my career. Although I had recently finished my master's degree, I was still craving the rigors and challenges of higher education and couldn't help fantasizing about giving up the fire department to pursue a different line of work. But I knew it would mean giving up all that I had worked for. So I would peruse the University of Central Florida's graduate catalog, trying to identify another degree program I could pursue alongside the fire department. I thought that if I could continue my education, perhaps I would be content with staying with the department and using my off-duty time to fulfill myself intellectually.

I had completed my BA in anthropology at the University of Central Florida, but the university had yet to implement a graduate program in this department. I considered a graduate degree in history, thinking it would be a fun and fulfilling way to occupy my free time, but what I really wanted was to study anthropology at the graduate level. Unfortunately, the closest program was in Gainesville at the University of Florida (UF). Gainesville is located about two hours north of Orlando. I knew the commute would be impossible, now that I was off shift and working a five-day workweek. As I vacillated between thoughts of leaving OFD and thoughts of continuing to pursue education on the side, I visited UF, meeting with the director of the CA Pound Human Identification Lab, the forensic anthropology lab located on the UF campus.

Forensic anthropology is the application of anthropological techniques (human skeletal analysis) in contemporary, legal contexts. It primarily deals with the identification of unknown persons and determining cause of death. The Pound Lab provides services for medical examiners and coroners throughout Florida. Its primary responsibility is to obtain the sex, age, and height of an unidentified person, along with any unique identifiers that would aid in the person's identification. The lab's second responsibility is to identify the cause of death of the individual, when possible.

Human remains are brought to the lab via law enforcement or, in cases requiring excavation, via forensic anthropologists or archaeologists who work in the lab. The remains arrive in various states of decomposition. Some are partially decomposed and arrive in body bags; others are fully skeletonized and have been in the ground or exposed for some time. I had developed a deep interest in forensic anthropology while completing my BA, reading numerous books on the subject. My years in the field of EMS had familiarized me with crime scenes involving dead bodies. Forensics afforded a link between anthropology and the type of scenes I encountered as a paramedic, and it felt like a natural extension of my work in EMS.

So I visited the lab and spent time with the director and some of his students, but compared to the field of EMS, the lab seemed like an oppressive atmosphere. I couldn't see myself being locked in a lab each day, surrounded by the remains of unknown individuals. I was used to spending much of my day outside in the elements, with a constant change of scenery. Hours of lab work held little interest for me. Ironically, I would return to the Pound Lab years later as a graduate student in order to hone my skills in trauma analysis of the human skeleton.

The program that really caught my eye was the graduate program in anthropology at Florida State University. FSU placed a heavy emphasis on archaeology within its program. It also provided a four-field approach to the study of anthropology, emphasizing the subfields of linguistics, cultural and physical anthropology, and archaeology. I had been to Tallahassee, a beautiful city of lush, rolling hills, very different from the flat landscapes of central Florida. I imagined myself living there, studying anthropology full-time, living a completely different life than I was living. These thoughts continually distracted me from the fire department.

I contacted one of the anthropology professors at FSU to discuss the program. At this point, I was approaching my ten-year anniversary at OFD. I knew I would become "vested" in my pension at that point and that if I was serious about pursuing a second career, this would be the time to do it. Having entered the field of EMS at the age of twenty-three, I was still young enough, even after a decade in the field, to switch careers.

My friends and family thought I was crazy. I had an excellent job, made a very comfortable living, had excellent benefits and job security, yet I was thinking about giving it all up to pursue a completely different course of study. But I couldn't put the thoughts out of my mind, so I applied. A few months later, I received a letter from FSU announcing my acceptance to the program. But in those few months, something happened that caused me to rethink leaving OFD: I took the district chief's promotional exam.

A FINAL STEP

When fire is burning out of a building and not affecting exposures, let it burn out and extend an interior attack from the unburned side. It is usually venting in the proper direction.

—OFD OFFENSIVE OPERATIONS

THE PROMOTIONAL EXAM FOR THE RANK OF DISTRICT CHIEF CAME around every two years. I was a lieutenant with ten years on the job, I had completed all the necessary coursework in addition to a master's degree and numerous advanced training courses, and I was obtaining administrative experience. If I was going to stay in the fire service, I was determined to be a chief.

District chiefs command a "district," or region within the city limits. There were three districts in Orlando at the time. I had spent the majority of my career in District 1, which covered most of downtown Orlando. Station 1, which housed Fire Administration prior to the building of Orlando's new City Hall, was the hub of the department and the place to be if you wanted to be in the middle of the action.

What I loved most about being at Station 1 was the close proximity to command. Here you could observe many administrative aspects of shift.

The division chief oversaw the entire shift. Under him were three district chiefs, or "districts," each responsible for his own region within the city. The districts typically oversaw three to four stations. Each lieutenant reported to a district chief, and administrative directives flowed up and down the chain of command.

The role of the district chief was one I had been eyeing for some time. I enjoyed being a lieutenant, especially when it came to managing crews on emergency scenes. But the districts were the ones who oversaw entire scenes. They took command upon arrival, deciding on the tactics to be utilized and generally controlling the flow of events as the scene unfolded. Administratively, they oversaw the stations within their district, making decisions about crew assignments, leave, and any disciplinary actions that cropped up.

They drove their own vehicles, so were free to roam the city as they pleased. I envied that freedom. As a crew member on an engine or rescue, errands required the participation of all members. As a firefighter, you had no say in the movement of your truck. It got better the higher you rose in rank. As lieutenant, you commanded your unit, but a good officer handled the minor decisions via consensus. Any errand-based truck movement became a "group thing."

I longed for the freedom of district chief. The thought of being able to spend each shift under my own itinerary sounded great. The thought of commanding fire scenes sounded even better. I had come to love the beauty and fluidity of fire-ground tactics. I excelled in my tactical training mainly because of my fascination with orchestrating effective tactics and controlling the complex logistics of emergency scene management.

I was also in the perfect position to sit for the promotional exam. I had done everything possible to prepare myself for the position of district chief and I wanted a shot at the promotion. Only one female in the history of the department had achieved the rank of district chief. She was one of the first females hired by the department, back when women were a truly rare commodity in the fire service. Her rise through the ranks had been a successful yet frustrating endeavor. She was educated and ambitious, a threatening combination for a woman in a man's field. But she persevered and ultimately obtained the rank of division chief, although the majority of her time as district and division chief was spent in administrative roles. This was no accident. Having a woman in charge of fire scenes was new to OFD, and many members of the department were not eager to take orders from a female. The general attitude seemed to be that she was more suited for an administrative position, as if the department were safer with her behind a desk rather than behind the wheel of a command vehicle.

A similar attitude permeated station staffing. Rarely were women assigned to the same station and shift. They were evenly distributed among stations and shifts, a practice spoken of openly among Administration. When I initially completed the hiring cycle for OFD, I was not hired with the first round of candidates. Appalled by the oversight, I contacted the deputy chief of the department, incensed that I was not picked up on the first round. Fortunately, he overlooked my insubordination and patiently explained that they "only needed to hire one female right now" and had decided on a female EMT instead of a female medic. He told me this casually, as if it was the norm within the department. I was too naïve at the time to be offended.

I was only the eighth female hired by OFD. Female acceptance among the men of the department was still a work in progress. I had kept my head down and worked hard, hoping for an easier path than my female predecessors. Although attitudes had improved dramatically over the years, females in charge were a source of contention among the men. I noticed little change in attitude when I was promoted to engineer. Engineers oversee the firefighters on their rigs, but their authority is limited by that of the lieutenant, who is ultimately responsible for the crew. But when I was promoted to lieutenant, I noticed subtle shifts in the attitudes of many members toward me.

The initial animosity seemed to stem from the ease with which I passed the exams. Each promotional exam results in a ranked list of candidates, from highest to lowest. Individuals are promoted based on their position on the list. On my engineer promotional exam, I scored number four out over thirty candidates. On the lieutenant's exam, I scored number six overall out of twenty-plus candidates, but obtained the highest score on the tactical portion of the exam. When the tactical scores were posted, some dismissed my score with "She's just a good test taker." The skeptics would do anything but admit that I was a proficient commander.

But after being promoted to lieutenant, it was if I had crossed some imaginary boundary. Suddenly I was considered a "climber," one who was only interested in achieving rank, which seemed ridiculous to me since all the candidates who sat for the exam were interested in achieving rank or they wouldn't have put themselves through the process. No one ever said firefighters were gifted with reason.

Following my promotion, my transition to the rank of lieutenant had been fairly uneventful, mainly due to the outstanding crew I was assigned: a seasoned engineer with a great sense of humor whom I had worked with for years and two newly hired, yet experienced firefighters who were more open-minded than most. But the transition wasn't free of conflict. There were subtle challenges to my authority on emergency scenes, mainly from firefighters questioning my directives; murmurs as I walked away after giving orders; and on occasion, firefighters actually asking me if I thought I was ready for the rank of lieutenant. It was galling, but part of the landscape. I was only the third female lieutenant in the history of the department, so I knew it would take time to be accepted. In no way did it deter me from going after the rank of district chief.

The promotional exam for district chief was like the lieutenant's exam on steroids. It consisted of three parts—a written exam that tested tactical knowledge and decision-making, an administrative exam, and a live tactical scenario. The written exam was complex but straightforward. The administrative exam was a three-part test: the candidate had to first manage an overflowing "In Basket" to test his or her ability to prioritize, plan, and make quick decisions; the second part involved counseling a problem employee; and the third involved teaching a class. For the teaching portion, candidates were presented a topic that they had to formulate into a coherent fifteen-minute class. The class was required to cover all necessary information in a comprehensive format, all the while dealing with a roomful of intentionally disruptive students. The disruptive students were those same role-players from the police department who participated in the lieutenant's exam, seasoned officers who possessed the attitudes and egos to convincingly portray obnoxious troublemakers. I aced the written and administrative portions of the exam. Now it was on to the live tactical scenario.

The tactical scenario was designed to simulate the pace and stress of a major emergency incident, a scene that ultimately goes down the toilet. The candidate sits in a district chief's command vehicle and gives all directives over the radio. The incident is designed to stress candidates and their resources beyond their capabilities; the vehicle and radio make the scenario as realistic as possible. I volunteered to go first.

The day of the exam, I arrived at my office as usual, since the scenario would play out on the training ground. The officers conducting the exam were located in one of the Training portables, radios in hand, ready to test the nerves and resolve of each candidate. A dispatcher was on site to handle radio traffic, and the entire scenario would be recorded. As I waited for the exam to begin, I went over tactics in my head, certain they would throw out the most complex of scenarios. I reviewed high-rise tactics, hazardous materials incidents, and mass casualty protocols. I felt ready for anything. Finally, one of the assessors entered the Training portable and told me to report to the command vehicle.

A district chief's Suburban was parked on the edge of the training ground. I climbed into the driver's seat, arranging my command paperwork next to me and setting my radio to the proper "tack" or channel. As soon as I was set, the radio came to life, dispatching multiple units to an apartment fire. I radioed my response and the scenario was on.

The assessors were made up of officers role-playing different unit commanders. As they each "arrived on scene," they radioed recon reports and their intended actions. The scenario was a multistoried apartment building with "heavy fire showing." As additional units arrived on scene, each officer reported his actions over the radio. The engine was pulling a 1¾" line; the "tower" was laddering the building to attempt rescue of victims on the second floor, since the fire had cut-off access via the stairwell; the second engine to arrive was pulling a backup line, and the rescue was treating patients on the ground. I made notes on my command worksheet of each unit, task, and each benchmark, waiting for the shit to hit the fan. It didn't take long.

Suddenly, one of the units reported that the fire had extended into the attic and was spreading the length of the structure. I redirected crews to enable a "stop" of the spread of fire and was surprised when they reported progress in attacking the fire. But then the "tower crew" reported they were cut off from the victims on the second floor and could make no further progress. I recommended having a second unit ladder the opposite side of the structure to gain access, but was quickly told they were unable to access the rear of the building. I could picture the officers huddled around their radios, giggling with delight as I wracked my brain to try to get my imaginary personnel to the imaginary victims.

I quickly realized this was the climax of the exam—risk versus gain! I had to make the decision to either continue to risk my personnel or resign myself to the fact that rescue of the victims was impossible. The scenario was quickly spiraling out of control, with multiple "units" reporting sagging of the roof and heavy fire. I advised the crew to vacate the structure and to switch to a "defensive mode." The imaginary crews evacuated the structure and reported that large-diameter hoses were being set up to fight the fire from the outside. The building, which by this time was fully involved with fire, was lost, and the victims left behind were charred. I was relieved to discover later that day that all the scenarios ended this way, some even worse.

By the end of the scenario, my heart was hammering in my chest, my stomach was in my throat, and I was so relieved I thought I would vomit. But I made it through and didn't kill any of my crew, which I felt confident would give me a few bonus points. I exited the vehicle, my legs weak and my hands still shaking, but thrilled to have it behind me. I returned to the Training portable to unwind and regroup, going over the scenario in my head and thinking how I could have handled it in retrospect. I knew the scenario would naturally devolve into chaos. That was the whole point of the test—to push candidates until they had to make a decision to pull the crews out and switch "modes," from an offensive to defensive attack.

It took another day and a half of testing to run all the candidates through. We then had to wait several days as scores were tabulated and the final list was compiled. I, however, was leaving town, heading to the Emergency Management Institute in Maryland. I was two days into my course when the call came; the list was completed. Out of twenty-plus candidates, I had come out number three, which guaranteed my promotion as soon as

I was eligible. Since I had only been a lieutenant for a year and a half, my promotion would be six months off. But I was on the list and on my way. I sat back, relishing the feeling of having performed well on the exam, thrilled at the thought of becoming a district chief.

But two issues weighed on my mind. The first was my acceptance to Florida State. Although I had worked extremely hard to succeed on the district exam, part of me still longed to pursue a career in anthropology. I had to make a decision concerning the graduate program in the next few weeks, a decision now compounded by my future as a district chief.

The second issue was being in the Training Division. I knew if I stayed with the department long enough to be promoted, I would need as much combat experience as possible, and I wasn't going to get it behind a desk. By the end of the two-week course at EMI, I had made my decision and drafted two letters: the first was to the chief of training, requesting a return to shift; the second was to Florida State, advising the Department of Anthropology I wouldn't be coming in the fall.

RETURNING TO SHIFT

Time becomes an extremely important factor with regard to attack operations. The bigger the attack or the more interior the attack is positioned, the longer it takes to get it going.

—OFD OFFENSIVE OPERATIONS

My request to return to shift was granted immediately and I returned to my original position on C Shift, District 1. I would be the District 1 "floating lieutenant," which meant I would be based out of Station 1 but "float" or "travel" within the district wherever a lieutenant was needed.

Many personnel don't like the position of floater. You are basically homeless; although you are assigned to a particular station, you may end up working anywhere in the city. Traveling from one station to another is no simple thing for a firefighter. Firefighters can't simply report to duty in uniform. They must bring with them all they will need for a twenty-four-hour shift. The most important piece of baggage is your gear, which includes bunker coat, pants, boots, hood, helmet, and any special equipment one chooses to wear with this gear. It might include personal escape equipment, tools, or specialized extrication gear.

Along with their gear, firefighters must also take their personal belongings. Most personnel carry a large duffle bad that contains all the personal items they will need for the shift: a change of uniform (for those scorching days when you sweat through your shirt before noon or those very special occasions when you are vomited on by a nauseous patient); personal hygiene gear, since it's tough to go a whole shift without showering; and anything else to make the shift pass quickly. Books, hobbies, and even auto repair equipment are part of the personal assemblages that are brought to the station for those evening hours when the chores are done and the calls have slowed.

The final piece of baggage is bedding. Each individual has his or her own set of bedding, most of it brought from home since the sheets and thin blankets provided by the department are no match for the subzero temperatures of the dorms. The beds within the dorm rooms are assigned and serve as the only private space each firefighter has. My space always included several must-have items: multiple pillows, since I spent much of the night reading and trying to fall back to sleep following each call; two lights—a reading light above my bed and a small flashlight for finding my way to the bathroom in the middle of the night; and the most important item—a turbo fan that sat above my head to drown out the sound of snoring that pervaded the dorm.

Dealing with snoring was one of the most challenging aspects of sleeping in a dorm full of men. The volume could be excruciating. There were a few members of the department known for their ear-splitting snoring. The worst offenders were banished to the "dayroom" (our term for the living area of the station). If they refused, they would invariably find their mattress and bedding relocated for them when they headed for bed.

I had served a stint as a floating engineer and had been forced to endure the snoring when I traveled to other stations. It was tough dragging my turbo fan with me everywhere, so I had to settle for a mini version, which was usually insufficient in drowning out the noise around me at night.

But floating as a lieutenant was a little better. The smaller stations, those that housed one or two trucks, typically had a private lieutenant's dorm that was separate from the main dorm. This was blissful. I loved finally having my own bedroom where I could read as long as I wanted without someone complaining about the light. The solitary quiet was a welcome relief after years of sleeping among the men.

Another aspect I appreciated about floating was the variation in crews, trucks, and locations. It's easy to become complacent with your crew, especially when it is a talented and experienced one. You develop a comfortable rhythm, each member knowing exactly what is expected at emergency scenes. Knowing the personalities of your crew is a great advantage when working within the intense atmosphere of fire and EMS. Over time, you can almost predict everyone's actions and how they will handle themselves, which makes for smooth-running scenes. As a floater, you may work with a different crew each shift. You can't rely on familiarity among crew members. You must always be alert to each individual's actions, since as the lieutenant, all of them are ultimately your responsibility. You must also develop flexibility and tolerance, since you may not always get along with those on your truck.

Familiarity with your truck is much the same. Most of the trucks are set up in the same format, so that if you need to retrieve equipment from someone else's truck on scene, you know where to go to get it. But each truck has small variations, depending on the year of manufacture and the personal preferences of the crews assigned. As a floater, you are forced to familiarize yourself with the layout of the truck each morning. This is vital to being able to act quickly on a scene and find what you are looking for. This constant refamiliarization is a great refresher in equipment and location on each rig. Again, there is little room for complacency.

Finally, I enjoyed working at different stations and different districts within the city. The change of scenery was a welcome relief from the routine of shift, and it gave me a chance to be exposed to many different types of buildings. When I was preparing for the engineer's promotional exam, I realized the best source of information and education was the seasoned members of the department. They had done and seen so much during their careers and were usually obliging in sharing what they had learned over the years. Whenever I was stationed with these personnel, I would tap their experience. They were the ones that knew the tricks of the trade.

My return to shift following the district chief's exam ushered in a new era in my career: I was now able to ride "out of grade" as a district chief. Since I had passed the promotional exam and had been a lieutenant for over a year, I was eligible to act as a district chief. My first shift riding out of grade was a nerve-wracking twenty-four hours.

I was to ride as District 1, which was a plus, since I knew the territory well and was familiar with the crews. That familiarity was also a challenge, since I would be commanding personnel (especially lieutenants) who still hadn't adjusted to my promotion to their rank. It was also a challenge being in a vehicle by myself, having to navigate without the aid of additional personnel to read the map. I was sure I would become terminally lost and end up wandering the city's streets in search of each call.

I was also nervous about having to command a major incident. One of the first calls of the day was an apartment fire. A full alarm was dispatched: a rescue, two engines, and a tower truck. I arrived on scene and radioed "District 1 assuming command," my first real-life experience in taking control of an emergency incident. It was awesome. I had my command sheet in hand, tracking the tasks of each unit and the flow of events. The fire was small and nearly out upon our arrival, but it still gave me the opportunity to try out the new rank on an actual emergency scene.

The remainder of the shift was uneventful. I responded to several other calls, but fortunately the city didn't burn down and I didn't total the district Suburban. All in all, it was a successful shift.

On the days when I stayed at Station 1, I had the opportunity to learn my way around the daily shift paperwork. Rosters had to be completed for the next shift, which meant rearranging personnel based on vacancies and individual skill levels. It was akin to a game of chess, with personnel and truck assignments as pawns. Empty slots on units had to be filled with individuals who were eligible to ride in those positions. Driver slots had to be filled with either engineers or relief drivers. At least one paramedic was required on each unit, since all the trucks within the department were certified for advanced cardiac life support (ACLS). Opportunities for riding "out of grade" were based on a rotation, so you had to ensure that these opportunities followed the proper order.

The months following my return to shift were filled with new experiences and responsibilities. I rode out of grade as a district chief on several occasions and was just starting to become comfortable in the role of command. I still experienced the occasional pang of yearning for graduate school. As September approached, I couldn't help but imagine what my life would have been like had I accepted the offer from Florida State. I would have been starting the graduate program, living in a new place with years of intense study ahead of me. Those thoughts became fantasy-like to me. I think everyone has those thoughts in the back of her mind: imagining leaving all she knows to venture out into a new world with new experiences. Or perhaps it was my transient upbringing that instilled in me the need for change, my abhorrence of routine.

Whatever it was, I fought through the urge to flee and remained focused on my upcoming promotion to district chief. My eligibility was a month away, retirements would be providing promotional opportunities, and I was learning everything I could about the responsibilities of my pending rank. Everything was in place for me to become the second female in the history of the department to make it to the rank of district chief. What I didn't know at the time was that the end of my career was just around the corner. The next months would be one of the most trying times in my life, when everything I had worked for was stripped from me and my future was forever changed.

PART FOUR

AND IT ALL CAME CRASHING DOWN

THE CALL

The decision to operate in a defensive mode indicates that the offensive attack strategy has been abandoned for reasons of personnel safety and the involved structure has been conceded as lost (written off).

—OFD DEFENSIVE OPERATIONS

Human memory is fallible. Our reactions within stressful situations can warp events as we recall them in our minds. What we remember as indisputable can later be proven false. Numerous court cases have shown that eyewitness testimony can be contradicted through DNA evidence.

I could recount for you the call that occurred on a morning in mid-August, a call that would set in motion events leading to the end of my career as a firefighter. But it would be limited to my perspective, my experience. So I have laid down this chapter using the official transcripts from radio transmissions. The transmissions are provided word for word. I have supplemented them with information to let the reader know what was happening between transmissions as the call unfolded.

For those not familiar with the staccato nature of radio communication on emergency scenes, it may be challenging to appreciate all that is happening amid the radio traffic. But radio traffic, especially on large-scale emergencies, is purposely kept to a minimum to avoid units talking over each other and to promote efficient communication.

I was the lieutenant on Engine 1 that day. The time frame provided in the transcripts that follow is the minutes and seconds elapsing from time of Dispatch's call. In the transcripts, "Unit" is the person or rig giving the radio transmission. "Dispatch" is the dispatcher on the radio; many of Dispatch's transmissions repeat information transmitted by each unit. "Radio Transmission" is what was actually said over the air. "107" is the radio designation for Division C, the division chief in charge of our shift who would take over command of the scene (a common procedure with large-scale incidents). In 2000, the computers within the OFD Dispatch Center could not identify the unit or radio giving the transmission as they can today (with the exception of emergency alert buttons located on individual portable radios); thus some transmissions are labeled "Unknown."

For logistical purposes, each structure on a fire scene has designated sides and quadrants. Side 1 is the front of the building and proceeds clockwise around the building, as Sides 2, 3 (back of the building) and 4. Quadrants mark the divisions inside the building, with quadrant A being the front left section of the building (when positioned in front, facing the structure), with quadrants B, C, and D going clockwise within the structure, dividing the inside of the building into four sections. These designations provide orientation for personnel working around and inside the structure. They also provide standard terminology when identifying a location within or outside of the building.

Alarm # 00-31629
Date of Call: 8/17/2000
Location: 1216 W. Washington St
Time of Call: 08:07 am

The call was dispatched at 8:07 A.M., just a few minutes following shift change. The first alarm was made up of two engines, a tower, a rescue, and a district chief. Due to the nature of the call and type of building, the division chief (Division C, also referred to as "107") responded.

Time	*Unit*	*Radio Transmission*
00:04	Division C	Division C responding.
00:14	E101	Engine 101 responding.
00:18	E7	Engine 7, Rescue 7 responding.
00:20	Dispatch	Engine 7, Rescue 7.
00:22	107	107's going to be responding to that call also.
00:24	Dispatch	107.
00:29	District 3	District 3 responding
00:30	Dispatch	District 3.
00:39	Dispatch	Tower 10 confirm response.
00:47	Tower 10	Tower 10 responding.
00:50	Dispatch	Tower 10 responding.
00:58	Dispatch	Orlando, District 3—we have received multiple calls reporting flames showing. We're dispatching Engine 1 and requesting Truck 30.

Additional units are automatically dispatched for large buildings with confirmed fire.

01:08	District 3	District 3 copy that.
01:11	Engine 1	Engine 1 responding.

I acknowledge responding as we clear a medical call at an assisted living facility downtown.

01:13	Dispatch	Engine 1.
01:15	501	501 will be responding.

"501" is the Training Chief, responding to act as Safety Sector.

01:16	Dispatch	501.
01:25	Engine 1	Engine 1 responding.

I repeated my response, perhaps not hearing Dispatch confirm my initial response.

01:26	Dispatch	Engine 1.
01:29	Inaudible	[Inaudible] to Orlando, give us a repeat on the address.
01:32	Dispatch	Unit calling you have low volume. This is Orange Blossom Trail and Washington.
01:36	Unknown	Check.
01:47	Engine 101	Engine 101 Orlando. How many alarms do you have coming to this?
01:51	Dispatch	Engine 101 repeat.
01:53	Engine 101	How many alarms do you have responding to the fire?
01:57	Dispatch	We've got a report that Tower 2 is on the scene requesting a 2nd alarm and Hazmat due to heavy explosives in the building. We are dispatching that now.

"Tower 2" was actually an off-duty lieutenant from Station 2 who had just left Station 2 and responded to the call in his personal vehicle. He has received the report of "heavy explosives in the building" from employees who have evacuated the building.

02:12	Engine 101	Engine 101 on scene. We have a transmission factory, heavy fire showing Side 1. We're going to investigate the building while pulling pre-connects. Second-in units bring us a line.

The report of heavy fire triggers a full second-alarm response, which is dispatched on the primary radio channel (thus the dispatch does not appear on this transcript). Engine 101 is asking for the next-in engine to bring in a supply line from the closest hydrant.

02:24	Dispatch	Copy Engine 1.
02:32	Unknown	101 I'm gonna need to get by you to get to the hydrant down behind you.
02:35	Engine 101	Check. I'm gonna be [inaudible] inside 3 of the building. There might be a better access. We got heavy fire, Side 1.
02:43	Engine 101	Engine 101, Engine 7.
02:48	Unknown	Inaudible.
02:56	Rescue 1	Rescue 1 responding.
02:58	Dispatch	Rescue 1.
03:00	Engine 3	Engine 3 responding.
03:01	Dispatch	Engine 3.
03:04	Tower 1	Tower 1 responding.
03:06	Dispatch	Tower 1.
03:12	Truck 30	Truck 30 responding.
03:15	107	107 on scene assuming command in front of the structure. Be advised—single story concrete block, heavy fire showing from the front.

Division C ("107") assumes command of the scene.

03:22	Dispatch	107 assuming command. Copy Truck 30.
03:26	Engine 101	Engine 101 to 107 we have been reported heavy fire in the front and the rear of the structure. We're pulling a 3 inch line due to the flammable liquid at this time.
03:45	District 2	District 2 on scene reporting to the command post.
03:49	Dispatch	District 2.
03:58	Engine 1	Engine 1 to Command. Do you have an assignment for us?
04:02	107	Command to Engine 1. Come on in and pull the second line off Engine 101.

04:11	Engine 101	Engine 101 to Command. We have about 2[00] to 300 gallons of flammable liquid inside many containers. I'm recommending that we go defensive on the building. We're gonna get a 3 inch line to the front door.

Engine 101's lieutenant is in charge of the Hazardous Materials Team (Haz Mat). He is recommending that the fire be fought from the outside, due to the heavy load of hazardous materials inside the building.

04:22	107	Command check. Command Orlando, be advised, be advised that this is going to be defensive until we get a knock down.

Per SOPs of defensive operations, page 2.13, Overview A: "The decision to operate in a defensive mode indicates that the offensive attack strategy has been abandoned for reasons of personnel safety, and the involved structure has been conceded as lost (written off)."

It is unknown why Command is suggesting a defensive mode until a knockdown is achieved. Knocking down the fire does not change the fact that there are heavy loads of hazardous materials inside the building. This would be the first of several breaches in OFD standard operating procedures.

04:29	Dispatch	Check.
04:36	Engine 101	Water on the fire.
04:38	Engine 1	Engine 1 on scene.

My unit arrives on scene and we proceed to pull a second 3" line off of Engine 101 and join the crew of Engine 101 at the front of the building (Side 1).

04:43	Dispatch	Copy Engine 1 and water on the fire.
04:45	Dispatch	This is a defensive mode. Repeating defensive mode.

Dispatch is alerting all units on scene that the fire is to be fought from the outside.

04:51	Engine 101	Engine 101 to Engine 101's Engineer, we have a straight tip line, give it water.
04:58	107	Command to Engine 101, be advised we've got 200 gallons of mineral spirits in the back of the building.

More hazardous materials are reported to bc inside the building, based on information from personnel who work in the transmission shop.

05:10	Engine 3	Engine 3 to Command. Would you like us to bring in a supply line?
05:16	107	Stand by for a minute Engine 3.
05:19	Engine 101	Engine 101 to Engine 101 Engineer. We got a straight tip line.
05:25	107	Command to Engine 3. Go one block south and see if you can make access to the back of the building.
05:35	Rescue 1	Rescue 1 to Command. Do you have an assignment?
05:39	107	Check. Rescue 1 come in to the scene and assist units.
05:45	Rescue 1	Rescue 1 check.
05:48	Haz Mat 1	Haz Mat 1 to Command. We're about 4 blocks away. Where do you want us?
05:53	107	Check. Just come to the front of the scene.
05:55	107	Command to Orlando. Be advised that we have water on the fire about two minutes ago.
06:00	Dispatch	Check, Command.
06:02	Rescue 1	Rescue 1 on scene. Side 4 of the structure.
06:05	Dispatch	Rescue 1.

06:08	Unknown	1 on the scene. Do you have an assignment Command?
06:12	107	Repeat unit on the scene.
06:13	Unknown	1. Requesting assignment.
06:16	107	Repeat unit number.
06:18	Tower 1	Tower 1. Tower 1.
06:22	107	Check, Tower 1. See if you can pull up in the front of Engine 101.
06:28	Tower 1	Copy. We'll pull up near [inaudible]. We're blocked by a line.
06:33	107	Check. See if you can go around the block, and come in from the other direction just in case we need to use your stick.
06:39	Tower 1	We're at Side 1. We'll cut through the parking lot here.

The building has perimeter fencing on both sides that extend to adjacent buildings. Therefore, crews are unable to walk from the front of the structure to the rear, without going around the entire block. Eventually, one of the tower crews cuts a hole in the fence to provide access to the rear of the structure.

06:43	Engine 101	Engine 101 to Command. We need a Tower truck to open some of these doors and windows on Side 1.
06:50	107	Command check. Tower 1 hold at that location and assist with forcible entry on the side.
07:07	102	102 responding.

"102" is the deputy chief of the department.

07:11	Dispatch	Was that 102?
07:13	102	Check.

07:16	District 2	District 2 to Command.
07:20	107	Go ahead District 2. Be advised that you will be Rear Sector.

By this time, District 2 has driven around the block to position his car on the back side (Side 3) of the structure. It is the first opportunity for any units to report conditions in the rear of the building due to the layout of the block and the perimeter fencing.

07:27	District 2	Copy. Rear Sector. Be advised that the building is shaped like a "U," opening in the center. You got the heavy involvement on Side 4. They are going to need to make the attack from Side 1 toward Side 4.

Despite the fact that the scene is in a defensive mode due to heavy loads of hazardous materials, District 2 is suggesting an interior attack.

07:41	107	Command check. Command to Sector, can you make entry into that front door on Side 1?
07:50	Unknown	Sir, they are attempting now.
07:54	District 3	District 3 on the scene, reporting to the Command vehicle.
07:59	Dispatch	District 3.
08:01	501	501 on the scene.
08:03	Dispatch	501.
08:12	Unknown	[Inaudible] to Command. Two minutes out.
08:16	107	Command check.
08:17	107	Command to 501. Upon arrival, go ahead and assume Safety Sector.

Safety Sector is responsible for monitoring the scene for conditions that would threaten the safety of crews, such as power lines and building integrity.

08:21	501	501 copy.
08:24	Engine 101	Engine 101 to Command. If you have the owner with you, what's the structure . . . do we have a second floor in here? And what's it loaded with?
08:32	107	Negative on the owner. I do not have the owner.
08:36	Engine 3	Engine 3 on the scene. Be advised, we have 55 gallon drums of brake fluid on the South side of the building. Chief, we're gonna need water. We're headed back to Central to get a plug.
08:53	107	Check Engine 3. Can you make access to the back via Central?
08:58	Engine 3	3 check. Chief, we have no water. We're going to Central. We have a open garage door back there with smoke pouring out of it.
09:06	107	Check. Go ahead and grab a plug and set up.
09:10	Engine 7	Engine 7 to Command. Do you need me to assist Engine 3?
09:14	Engine 1	Engine 1 to Command. We have a [inaudible] . . . fire inside of the structure. We have oil involved on the middle of the structure.

This is my broken radio transmission where I am advising Command that there is heavy fire on the second floor. I can see the second-floor involvement from my position at the front bay door of the building. I can also see large pools of burning oil in the center of the first floor. Command does not acknowledge my transmission.

09:24	Truck 30	Truck 30 on scene.
09:27	Dispatch	Truck 30.

09:30	Engine 101	Engine 101 to Command. I'll let you know when to pump my plug. I'm down at 100 on my vacuum.
09:36	107	Command check. Command to Engine 7. Can you pump Engine 101's plug?
09:43	Engine 7	Engine 7 check.
09:46	Haz Mat 1	Haz Mat 1 on the scene.
09:49	Dispatch	Haz Mat 1.
09:53	Engine 3	Engine 3 to Command. We're laying in one 4 inch supply line from Central and Wilson. We're gonna operate a large diameter line from the rear.
10:06	107	Command check.

At this point, Command is allowing opposing hand lines to be placed in operation—two lines are operating at the front of the building, and he has just acknowledged that Engine 3 will be operating a line from the rear of the structure. Opposing hand lines should never be allowed to operate on a fire scene.

10:07	107	Command to Engine 3. Do you need additional help?
10:13	Engine 3	We will, Chief, when we get a supply line laid. We're a couple minutes away from that.
10:20	District 2	Rear Sector to Command.
10:24	107	Go ahead Rear.
10:26	District 2	On Side 3, we got both bay doors open. It looks like they had a fire knock down, coming in from you Side 1, quadrant D. We need to get a line in here from Engine 3 and attack this from the rear side. We got both doors open. We can make an easy attack from the rear, Side 3.

District 2 is again recommending an interior attack. Although the fire near the front of the structure on the first floor has been knocked down, the building still contains heavy loads of hazardous materials. Command has already advised Engine 101 that there are 200 gallons of mineral spirits at the rear of the building, per information from warehouse employees. District 2 is unaware of the heavy involvement on the second floor, since the stairwell is located near the front of the structure and is not visible from the rear of the building.

10:45	107	Command check. They are in the process of laying a line. Can you re-assign someone to assist to set up a large diameter line in back with them?

The instruction by 107 to set up a large diameter line implies they will continue to operate defensively.

10:58	Tower 10	Tower 10 on the scene.
11:00	Dispatch	Tower 10.
11:02	501	Safety to Command. Are we still in a defensive mode?
11:06	701	Command check.
11:10	District 2	Rear Sector to Command. Be advised, we've got no fire on Side 3. We've got both bay doors open. Quadrants A, B, and C and D. We can make an offensive attack on this. We'll need to hold the Side 1 attack and come Side 3, rear attack sector. We need to assign additional units to my side, Rear Sector. All I have is Engine 3.
11:34	107	Command check. Command to Safety. Have people move from under those power lines. We just had one that fell.

11:41	501	Check. Also, you have interior operations going on, on Side 1. You need to pull those people out.

Despite the scene being in defensive mode, Engine 7's crew had made entry via the front of the structure.

11:48	107	Check. Will you go through and have them pull out please?
11:53	501	Command check.
11:56	Engine 7	Engine 7 to Command. We copy. We're backing out.
12:01	107	Command check.
12:11	107	Command to Rear Sector.
12:15	District 2	Rear Sector to Command.
12:18	107	Were you able to re-assign somebody to assist Engine 3?
12:23	District 2	Rear Sector to Command. Be advised, I'm with the owner. He advised that both these bay doors on the East and West sides, we can walk all the way through with blinds and knock this fire out. We need to make the attack from the Rear Sector. Assign me additional units to back up Engine 3. Got a 1¾" coming in.

At this point, District 2 is sending in a single engine company with a small hand line. It is against SOPs to send an engine company into a commercial structure without a backup line in place in the form of a second crew with an additional hand line for protection. The two lines are to enter the structure simultaneously. It is also questionable to fight a commercial fire with small hand lines that are typically reserved for house or car fires.

12:41	107	Check. We have Tower 30 on the scene. Would you like to use them?
12:52	Dispatch	Orlando to Command. The building owner, a Louis Cassel, is on the scene.
12:58	Rescue 1	Rescue 1. Utilities controlled.
13:04	107	Command check. Rescue, 1, utilities controlled. Rescue 1 take your personnel and assist Engine 3 on the back side of the building, please.
13:15	Engine 7	Engine 7 to Orlando we're on Side 4 of the building with Tower 1 outside Team.
13:23	District 2	Rear Sector to Command. Who did you assign me and Engine 3? I have Tower 1 and Engine 3. Correct, Tower 10 and Engine 3.
13:30	107	Check. You'll have Rescue 1 also assigned to you.
13:36	District 2	Check. I want to avoid opposing attack lines. If I can get another crew back here to do two lines attacking from the rear sector, not from Side 1.
13:45	107	Check. There is no line flowing in the front at this time.

At this point, my crew and Engine 101's crew had shut down our lines at the front of the structure and were changing out our air bottles.

13:50	District 2	Check. I need another engine company for a back-up line.
14:00	107	Check.
14:02	District 2	Also confirming that we have a RIT team, need a RIT team on standby, rear sector.

A RIT team is a Rapid Intervention Team.

14:07	107	Check. We have Tower 30 as a RIT.
14:15	Engine 101	Engine 101 to Command. We have a [inaudible] the fire on Side 1 knock-down, except for a couple of hotspots. Do you still want us to operate on Side 1?
14:25	107	Check 101. Hold your position on Side 1.
14:34	Engine 3	Engine 3 to 3 Driver. Charge the 1¾".

Engine 3 is having its driver charge its hose line. Charging the line is done just prior to making entry into a structure.

14:40	107	Command to Chief Dickens. Report back to the Command Post.
15:00	District 2	Rear Sector. Advise the secondary backup engine you got coming.

District 2 knows that he should have a backup line in place prior to Engine 3 entering the building.

15:06	107	Stand by at this time.
15:14	District 2	Rear Sector to Command. Be advised, I got 2 from Tower 10, Rescue 1 crew—2 men, Engine 3—3 men. They can attack interior, working off of Side 3, quadrant B, working around to A, and around to D and C. Full circle.
15:32	107	Command check. Do you got a back-up line, and initial attack line?
15:36	District 2	Negative. I'm waiting for assignment of a crew for a back-up line and an engine crew around to the rear.

District 2 admits that he has no backup line in place but has already sent in the interior crews.

15:43	107	Command check. We're changing out some bottles. As soon as we get some bottles changed out we'll send someone around.
15:49	District 2	Check. Be advised, we got a tag line on the search team, and a hand line on Engine 3 crew.
15:56	107	Check. Command to Engine 1.

Command is contacting me to order me and my crew to the rear of the building. I was in close proximity to the command vehicle, so I walked over and he gave me the order face to face.

16:07	102	102 to Orlando. I've been on the scene about 4 minutes. I'm at the Command Post.
16:11	Dispatch	102.
16:14	502	Safety to Command. As soon as we can, let's find out what an ETA on OUC [Orlando Utilities Commission] and let us know when power gets shut to the building.
16:24	Engine 7	Engine 7 to Command. [Inaudible] to the Y-line, and where you need us to run it to.
16:30	107	Check, Engine 7. Hold your position in front of the building, do not spray any water.
16:37	Engine 7	Check.
16:40	District 2	Rear Sector to Command. If you have a crew, ready to go, i.e. Engine 7, send them

		to the rear so we can get a back-up line in with Engine 3.

Again, District 2 is requesting a crew to back up Engine 3. By this time, crews have been inside the structure for two minutes with no backup line in place.

16:49	107	Command to Rear Sector. Be advised, you'll have Engine 1 assist with the back-up line. They are en route to your location at this time.

My crew and I tried to make it to the rear of the structure via Side 4 but were cut off by the fence. We then circled back around the front of the structure and were able to make it through the cut fence on Side 2.

16:57	District 2	Rear Sector check. Have we got a Truck company to the roof to give us a report?

On a commercial structure fire, a tower truck is supposed to set up and provide an assessment of roof conditions as soon as possible.

17:03	107	Stand by. Command to Tower 1.
17:08	Tower 1	You got Tower 1, go ahead. We got the rest of Side 1 open, we're gonna proceed around to the back side. If you need a truck, I don't know where the second one is.
17:16	107	Check. Are you able to put up a ladder on the corner of the wall and give me a report from the roof?
17:23	Tower 1	Copy. You need a report of the roof?
17:27	107	Command check.
17:30	Dispatch	Orlando to Command. OUC's ETA—10.

17:37	107	Command to Rear Sector. Be advised, we do have fire through the roof on Side 4, quadrant . . . correction, quadrant B.
17:53	District 2	Confirming, Side 1, quadrant D—as in dog?
17:59	107	That's affirmative. We do have fire through the roof.

Command can see fire through the roof from his location near the front of the structure. The fire through the roof is coming from the heavy fire on the second floor. District 2 is still unaware that there is heavy fire on the second floor. Once fire has penetrated a roof, the entire roof structure can become unstable, especially in large commercial structures.

18:08	District 2	Check. Keep me advised, I got a crew, deep in, going in Area C into A, and working their way around to D. Keep me advised of conditions.

District 2 is confirming that he has crews deep inside the building, still with no backup line in place. He makes no move to order crews out of the structure, even with the report of fire through the roof.

Structural Collapse SOP, page 5.5, D: "In a typical fire involved building, the roof is the most likely candidate for failure, however, failure of the roof may very likely trigger a collapse of one or more wall sections."

18:18	107	Command check. Also, we had some old gas lines, natural gas lines, running through the building. Do you know if there is a gas meter on the back side?
18:33	Engine 7	Engine 7 to Command. We're free. Do you want us to pull a hand line to the rear of the structure?
18:40	107	Engine 1 is doing that. [Inaudible.]
18:45	Engine 7	Check.

18:52	District 2	Rear Sector to Engine 3. Give me a report.
18:57	Engine 3	Engine 3 to Rear Sector. We've knocked down a small amount of fire. We're making our way to where the first fire attack was made. We have very little fire at our location.

The fire on the first floor had been knocked down by the initial attack from the front of the structure. Engine 3 has yet to make it to the second floor.

19:13	Dispatch	Engine 1 left jump, advise your condition.

By accident, my firefighter had activated his emergency button on his portable radio.

19:20	Dispatch	Orlando to Engine 1, advise your condition, Engine 1, left jump.
19:26	Engine 1-L/J	Accidental Orlando.
19:29	Dispatch	Check. Turn off your radio off and back on to reset.
19:33	District 2	Rear Sector to Command. Need a report on the roof condition, fire conditions on Side 1.

District 2 is concerned about roof conditions, especially with crews making an interior attack.

19:45	107	Command to Tower 1. Hey Pete, have you checked the roof yet?
19:55	Tower 1	Check. We're on the way right now.
19:59	107	Check. As soon as you get it, let Rear Sector—District 2—know.
20:05	Tower 1	Copy.

It is at this point that my crew and I arrive at the rear of the structure. I see that there is a hose line snaking into the building and am sure there has been a breakdown in communication, since I was unaware that the fire had shifted to an offensive (interior) attack. There was no radio transmission declaring a switch from defensive to offensive mode, and I was under the impression that I was reporting to the Rear Sector to pull a backup, exterior line for Engine 3, as we had done for Engine 101.

District 2 approaches me and orders me to pull a backup line and enter the building to back up Engine 3. He then walks away. I'm unable to comprehend why there are crews inside when there have been multiple reports of hazardous materials within the building, all employees of the transmission shop have been evacuated, and we have been working in a defensive mode at the front of the structure.

I approach District 2 and advise him that we have been fighting the fire in a defensive mode. He makes no reply, but orders me again to back up Engine 3. He then walks away again before I can respond.

20:09	107	Command to Rear Sector. Also be advised that we haven't been set up in the front of the building.

Command is warning District 2 that they have yet to obtain a clear picture of the extent of fire on the roof or the conditions of the roof, since a tower truck has yet to set up in front of the building.

20:16	District 2	I copy. I want to re-remind you, I got Engine 3 company deep seated, they are probably at Side 1 working their way toward C. They say they don't have any heavy fire, but I'm still seeing a lot of smoke from D, can you give me a report?
20:28	107	Check. There still is some fire coming through the roof. I don't see any coming

		from inside. It could be just a roof fire at this point.
20:35	Engine 3	Engine 3 to Rear Sector. We're poised at the stairwell to go to the second floor. I feel heat up here. There may be fire on the second floor.

Engine 3 is confirming my earlier radio transmission of fire on the second floor.

20:48	Tower 10	Tower 10—outside to Command.

I hold up my index finger to my firefighter, indicating to wait before entering and I approach District 2 for the second time. I advise him I have seen heavy fire on the second floor from Side 1 and that he needs to pull the interior crews out. We are both yelling to be heard over the noise of Engine 3, which is parked just behind us. He yells back, telling me he is giving me an order to back up Engine 3, pointing to the opening in the rear of the building with his radio. I yell back that he has not seen conditions from Side 1, as I have, and that we should be operating in a defensive mode. I urge him to get a report from Engine 3 from inside the structure. He walks away from me and then radios Engine 3, asking for a situation report.

21:00	District 2	Engine 3, report your location and your condition.
21:05	Engine 3	Engine 3 to Rear Sector. We are poised to make an entry to the second floor from the stairwell in the interior. Is this now a defensive attack?

Engine 3 is unsure whether to proceed to the second floor.

21:19	District 2	Be advised . . . Rear Sector, Command. Make this a defensive operation. Back all

units out. At this point we have Tower 10—2 men, Rescue 1—2 men, 3 men on Engine 3.

After hearing the report from Engine 3, District 2 decides to return to defensive mode and pull out all interior crews.

21:38	Tower 1	Tower 1 to Command. The first entry spot that Engine 101 made, there is a partial roof sagging in that area. The rest of the structure, the roof structure looks sound—all but that first attack area.
21:51	107	Command copy. Command to Rear Sector. Did you copy? Side 1, quadrant D—sagging. We still got another fire on the roof.
22:01	District 2	Check. Engine 3's reporting they are on the second floor, on Side 1, looks like quadrant A headed to D and getting heavy fire on the second floor.
22:11	107	Check. Command to Rear Sector. Do we need to back out and go back to a defensive mode?

Command is unaware that District 2 has already suggested returning to defensive mode.

22:20	District 2	Rear Sector to Engine 3. Give me a report of your condition.

Although District 2 has already advised Command to return to a defensive mode, he questions Engine 3 again as to their condition.

22:25	Tower 1	Tower 1 to Command. The roof on Side 1, quadrant B is starting to sag. It's starting

		to bow out. Side 1, where we made entry has got a small crack in it. It's starting to bow outward. Be aware of crews working in that area.
22:39	Tower 10	Tower 10 to Command. I have Engine 3 handjacking us a line for aerial ops if needed.
22:45	107	Command check. Command to Rear Sector. Did you copy Tower 1? We do have roof sag in the front now. You may want to back Engine 3 and inside crews out.
22:54	District 2	Check. We have Engine 3 out. Make an account for all personnel. We'll go defensive operation.
23:00	107	Command check.

The altercation I had with District 2 took less than two minutes. He advised Command to switch back to a defensive mode immediately after I suggested he obtain a condition report from Engine 3, who also asked him if we were now in a defensive mode.

Once the scene had officially returned to a defensive mode, large diameter hoses were set up outside the structure and water flowed for another two hours until the fire was out.

I didn't think much about the altercation with District 2. I felt there had been a breakdown in communication and that District 2 had been working independently of the rest of the scene. I also felt he was aggravated that he was forced to follow my recommendation to pull crews out as the situation deteriorated.

On a large-scale fire scene, it is difficult to monitor all radio conversations, even though we try. Because we were working large-diameter streams at the front of the structure, the noise levels inhibited radio traffic, and it was difficult to follow all communications between Command and District 2. There was no dispatch notification that the mode of fire was switching to an interior attack. I was working off the information I had initially received on scene concerning the heavy loads of flammable and explosive materials and the fact that there was no life hazard, since all employees of the transmission shop were accounted for. Having seen the heavy fire within the main area of the structure when working from Side 1, I knew the building's integrity was compromised and that one of the potential dangers of large open buildings impacted by fire is collapse. I felt every second counted in getting interior crews out.

As for my actions toward District 2, I knew I had been forceful in my argument, but I felt the urgency of the situation necessitated it. The noise level on scene was high so it was natural that our voices were raised. My demeanor was definitely aggressive. It was impossible for me to remain passive when confronted with what I believed were contradictory and dangerous tactics on scene.

As operations continued, I interacted with District 2, setting up a large diameter line per his orders. Nothing more was said between us about the altercation, and I believed it to be behind us. I had been on previous fire scenes were personnel butted heads over tactics; not that arguing orders was common place, but our SOPs clearly stated that it was the responsibility of fire officers to bring to the attention those commanding the scene any potentially dangerous situations.

My biggest concern had been the safety of interior crews. At the time, I didn't know how many of our personnel were inside the structure; I was just determined to see that they were removed. Had I known that there were six people inside, I probably would have been even more aggressive in persuading him to switch tactics.

When we returned to the station following the call, I was still going over the events in my head. I pulled my engineer, Scott, aside, curious about his take on my run-in with District 2, since Scott was a seasoned veteran and had been standing close by when the altercation occurred. I asked him what went through his mind when we came around the rear of the structure and saw that there were firefighters inside.

He replied, "All I could think of was Worcester."

On a cold December night in 1999 in Worcester, Massachusetts, six firefighters were killed in a large warehouse fire after they became lost in heavy smoke and ran out of air. The fire was started by homeless people living within the building. It took five days to put the fire out, eight to find the bodies of the firefighters. The incident underscored the dangers involved in large commercial structure fires.

Scott closed our discussion with, "The last thing I wanted to do was enter that building."

I felt reassured that I was not alone in my concerns over the tactics and safety of crews at the scene. He told me not to worry about it and joked that District 2 would get me back at some point down the road.

I also spoke with JJ, the lieutenant in charge of Engine 101 and the Haz Mat Team. The first thing he said to me when I sat down with him in the dayroom was, "No one ever should have been in that building."

It wasn't until later in the day that I started catching hints of gossip concerning the altercation. I wasn't aware that anyone had paid any attention to it, so caught up was I with the situation on scene. But as the day wore on and we discussed the call, a few of the firefighters started asking me questions. I brushed the incident off as a misunderstanding, stating that there were communication issues on scene typical of large-scale incidents. Then I was called into the division chief's office.

As I entered the office, the division chief, my district chief, and District 2 were already inside. I could tell they had been having a heated discussion; District 2 shot me an icy look as I entered. My division chief, an excellent commander and good-natured individual whom I had worked with my entire career, opened the conversation by stating that he felt my conduct on the scene had been too assertive. He understood that I was looking out for the safety of the crews involved, but that I should have handled it with greater tact.

Considering the fact that I felt District 2's actions were risking the lives of the interior crews, I argued, I felt I had communicated with appropriate urgency to get my point across. The division chief tried to diffuse the matter by stating that there had obviously been a lack of communication on the scene, since I was unaware the scene had switched to an offensive attack. I reminded him that the declaration had never been made over the radio and that when I arrived at the rear of the structure, I felt sure that opposing hand lines were being utilized (an unsafe tactic where the fire is attacked from opposite directions). I said that it was my responsibility to pass on the information concerning heavy fire on the second floor and it was my belief that District 2 had jeopardized the lives of the crews by deploying an interior attack.

As the conversation continued, I became more frustrated and District 2 became angrier. We started arguing about the tactics on scene. District 2 asserted that I had risked the interior crews by not immediately backing them up. I argued that had he been so concerned about a backup line, he should have followed SOPs and not sent in the crews without a backup line already in place. The division chief finally halted the discussion after I accused District 2 of being pissed off because he had had to do exactly as I advised—pull the crews out and return to a defensive mode.

District 2 was furious. The conversation had devolved to a yelling match and once again, the division chief tried to calm us down, stating that he believed my intentions were good, but that I should monitor my radio more closely on scenes and handle similar situations less aggressively. It was obvious he wasn't going to discuss the tactics on scene, since he had been in command and had allowed District 2 to pursue the interior attack.

I left the room, feeling the ass-chewing I received would be the last of it and that I had probably made an enemy of District 2. My division chief assured me later that evening that it would blow over, that my intentions were good, but that I had to be careful who I went up against, since some chiefs didn't appreciate being advised by subordinates on scenes.

I felt confident that as things cooled down, we would move past it and put it behind us. I was a month away from being promoted to district chief and didn't want enemies in the ranks, so I sent District 2 an email the next day apologizing for my aggressiveness on scene, but stating again that I was acting on behalf of the safety of the crews, both interior and my own, and that I would try to use greater tact in the future.

I believed that was the end of it. I felt the apology would help diffuse the situation, since we had had a good working relationship prior to the incident. What I didn't realize was his level of anger at having been directed on scene in front of other personnel, the fact that rumors were already spreading furiously through the department about the incident, and that others were urging him to "teach me a lesson" about following orders on emergency scenes. My rank and future were about to be placed on the line.

CHARGES

Command should abandon marginal attacks when it is determined that the roof is unsafe, or when interior forces encounter heavy heat and cannot locate the fire or cannot make progress on the fire.

—OFD OFFENSIVE OPERATIONS

THE DAYS FOLLOWING THE INCIDENT WERE FILLED WITH INNUENDO. Many of my coworkers approached me, asking me what had happened on scene. I continued to downplay the incident, not wanting to fuel the rumor mill. But behind the scenes, District 2 was lining up forces against me. I found out a few days later that the off-duty lieutenant who had been on the scene of the incident, the same one that advised Dispatch of "heavy explosives in the building," was now urging District 2 to charge me with insubordination, since I did not automatically enter the structure on his command. His hypocrisy was just a tip of the iceberg of what I would encounter as the month went on.

District 2 held a private meeting with the commander of our Special Investigative Services (SIS) to decide which codes of conduct I had violated on scene. He intended to go after me with as many violations as possible, even if the violations overlapped. The fact that the chief of SIS was assisting him was the first of many unorthodox steps in the process of prosecuting me, especially considering the fact that he was due to retire in a few months and had not been taking on new cases. He had decided not to pass my case to his next-in-command. Whether this was due to the nature of the case or his long history of pursuing charges against female employees is unknown.

They decided I would be charged on three counts: insubordination, failure to obey, and failure to assist. It didn't seem to matter that insubordination and failure to obey were basically the same charge. District 2 wanted as many counts as possible on the paperwork, perhaps to make the incident appear more serious that it actually was. Whether he was fueled by his own anger or was simply being peer-pressured into charging me, I will never know. Perhaps it was a combination of both.

Prior to the incident, he and I had had a good working relationship. As I was learning the ropes of district-level administration, I sought his counsel on basic tasks such as developing shift rosters and managing administrative paperwork. He had always provided useful information with no hint of animosity toward me.

District 2 had a reputation as a focused administrator and an exceptional fire officer. I had always admired his composure and drive. He was polished and professional, one of the rising stars of the department, which is why I turned to him when I had administrative questions. I knew he took a thoughtful, meticulous approach to managing his district and I wanted to emulate those characteristics.

I thought back to a previous incident, just a few weeks before the warehouse fire, when I had been in the division chief's office with my district chief and District 2, discussing departmental politics and various aspects of administration. I remember looking around the room, excited about the caliber of officers I now interacted with, since my two-year anniversary as a lieutenant was quickly approaching, as was my promotion to district chief. I felt pride in the fact that, like them, I had aggressively pursued every aspect of higher education. I had completed a master's degree; I had attended some of the most elite tactical schools; and I had an excellent work history within the department. In my nearly eleven years with OFD, I received only minor disciplinary reprimands, I rarely used sick time, and I had never once been late for duty. I felt immune to any serious disciplinary action, since I had always been a conscientious employee.

But things were happening behind the scenes and there would be little I could do to slow them down.

A GATHERING STORM

Beware of "Crisis Management" where the situation grows at a rate faster than the response to that situation—Command ends up with an out of control situation and inadequate resources to control it.

—OFD ADDITIONAL RESOURCE MANAGEMENT

I WAS FORMERLY CHARGED WITHIN A FEW DAYS. MY DIVISION CHIEF, who served as Command on the scene, was as surprised as me. He had assured me things would blow over and that District 2 was merely angry. But things didn't blow over; they quickly spiraled into a major incident.

I met with Mark, one of the union representatives, soon after the charges were filed. In spite of the charges, I still believed the incident could be handled quietly and quickly—that I would get time off without pay to set an example for other personnel and to provide District 2 a means of saving face. Mark and I sat down in one of the offices at Station 1 and the first thing he said was, "I think we can save your job."

I thought he was kidding. I looked at him, stunned, not believing what I was hearing. I gave him an abbreviated account of the incident: how shocked I was when I came around the building to see an interior attack being fought; how I confronted District 2 about the fact that we had been fighting an exterior attack at the front of the building; that there was heavy fire on the second floor, and that he needed to remove interior crews. I explained to Mark that immediately following our verbal confrontation on scene, District 2 had radioed interior crews, who backed up everything I had told him. They reported fire on the second floor and questioned if the scene had returned to a defensive mode. District 2 had immediately ordered the crews to evacuate and return to a defensive mode, which seemed to justify my confrontation and questioning of his tactics.

I told Mark the whole encounter took about two minutes and that there was no way I should lose my job over carrying out my responsibilities as an officer. I told him about District 2's anger over the incident and that he was just pissed off for having to follow my advice. I also told Mark that as a union representative, he needed to try to cool things down within the department, that the gossip was turning the incident into a witch hunt, and that, as a union officer, he needed to set the example and downplay the event. Mark seemed reluctant to commit to my defense. We had been friends a long time, having been hired together. His reticence was the first of many such encounters I would have with union reps and members of my department.

I had seen this type of thing happen in the department before, the playing up of minor incidents. It was as if members needed a good story every so often to keep things interesting. When a good story didn't materialize, they would blow an incident out of proportion, just to have something to talk about. It was like a slow news day among the cable networks. When there's nothing to report, suddenly minor stories are given maximum airtime, just to give the talking heads something to chew on.

I was scared. My private life had always been a source of gossip around the department and I was familiar with the ferocity of the rumor mill. Even when I was initially hired, there were rumors about my background, where I had come from, and what I did with my free time. I lived a different lifestyle than most of the members of the department. The majority of the members lived typical middle-class lives—a nice house in the suburbs, a spouse, and kids. They kept up with the events of each other's lives by comparing notes on their children—what grades they were entering, what accomplishments they made in school, how old the kids were getting. I could never understand the draw of settling down and having children. To me it was anathema to everything I wanted for my future.

I had decided early on that I would never have children. The thought of my life revolving around the needs of kids never attracted me. I also felt no need to get married. I had been married briefly early in my career to an ambitious and respected police officer who worked for the Orlando Police Department. But we had very different ideas about what we wanted for our future. He came from a tight-knit family and wanted children. My goals had never included kids, so we parted after two years of marriage, both content to go our separate ways.

I kept to myself on my days off. I typically didn't involve myself with a lot of departmental activities. As a female, I always felt that I was intruding on "guy time" when I attended union meetings or hung out with groups from the department. Not that I didn't socialize among the department. But as I got older, especially after being promoted to lieutenant, I felt more out of place and less inclined to get involved in departmental activities.

The fact that I chose to remain single didn't help matters. I was constantly asked when I was going to "settle down" and have kids, as if it was a required step in one's life. But I had no intention of ever having kids and had already had a tubal ligation. I loved my simple life of reporting to duty, working, and having a wealth of time off to attend classes, workout, and travel. I couldn't imagine changing my life from its easy pace.

My relationship status seemed a constant source of gossip among my shift. Why it mattered to anyone, I'll never know. I never delved into my coworker's private lives and really didn't feel compelled to know who they were sleeping with, but for some reason, my social life (or sometimes the lack thereof) was frequently discussed. If I spent any time at all with any one of my coworkers, it was automatically rumored that I was sleeping with them. I had a few friends I would hang out with. We would play racquetball, go to movies, and even travel together. But they were platonic relationships, which were never understood or accepted by my coworkers. I used to joke that if I had actually slept with every person rumors connected me with, I never would have had time to go to school.

There were relationships that went beyond friendship. I know the old adage "Don't shit where you eat," which is a wise rule to live by. But for a single female working within a male-dominated field among young, aggressive males, it was a hard rule to abide by. I was intensely private about my personal life. I felt it was no one's business and I never let it affect my work performance or ambitions. But the double standard that exists concerning males and females and their sexual partners is even more rigid within male-dominated fields.

I didn't care. I lived my life as I wanted and wasn't concerned about what people said about me, true or false. I learned early on that if I fretted over every rumor, I would have a long and painful career. So I ignored their petty gossip and did as I pleased, which only seemed to fuel the mill.

But now the rumor mill was grinding away, not about my personal life, but about my actions on the job. This was new territory for me. I had always been extremely cautious about checking out my truck and equipment; I compulsively completed paperwork after each call, never putting it aside for later. I loathe procrastination. Following my promotion to lieutenant, I was even more cautious about maintaining a professional demeanor on duty so that I would be looked on as a respectable officer.

Now my conduct as an officer was in question and the rumors surrounding the incident were becoming more implausible by the day. People were saying that I had blatantly refused an order on scene, that I had had a screaming match with District 2, that I had thrown down my gear in a huff, refusing to enter the building—ridiculous accounts of a situation that should have been handled by those involved on scene, not by the whims of public opinion among the department.

I urged Mark to speak to the union board and squash the rumors concerning the incident. I could feel the weight of negative opinion building and I was scared. This was how reputations were ruined—by incidents on emergency scenes that were inflated by rumor and turned into urban myths among the department. It was especially true for females in the department. Our actions were always overscrutinized. When there were incidents, it was always the women that were made into the neurotic, unreasonable individuals, no matter who was really at fault. I knew I was getting sucked into a losing battle.

"They've got me," I thought, as Mark and I parted. My promotion to district chief was quickly approaching, which intensified the gravity of the situation. I knew being found guilty on the charges would risk my promotional status, but up until that point, I had never thought seriously that the situation would go this far. Suddenly, everything was caving in and I felt incapable of stopping it. It would only get worse.

VERDICT

Some tactical situations move slowly, while some move very quickly. Command must call for additional resources at a rate that stays ahead of the fire.

—OFD ADDITIONAL RESOURCE MANAGEMENT

THE INVESTIGATION BEGAN AND SOME OF THOSE WHO HAD BEEN ON scene were interviewed. I felt confident that since District 2's charges stemmed from my lack of putting the backup line into operation, eventually someone would get around to asking why the first crews were sent in without the backup line in the first place. But the question was never raised. In fact, none of the tactics were ever reviewed or questioned.

It wasn't until the investigation was completed that I would learn of my coworkers' lack of support when it came to my actions on scene. Even my engineer, who had told me the first thing that came to mind when we approached the rear of the building was the deaths at Worchester, changed his tone when questioned by SIS. When asked about my demeanor on scene, he responded, "She had fear all over her face"—nothing about his own concern based on the tactics being utilized, nothing about the safety of interior crews. But then again, he had no opportunity to add his own perspective of the scene itself; he was never asked about it.

SIS was careful about who was interviewed and which questions were asked. For some reason, major players were left out of the investigations. The first-arriving lieutenant, leader of the Haz Mat Team who first advised Command to perform an exterior attack due to heavy loads of hazardous materials in the building, was never interviewed. And the questions posed to my division chief, who had served as Command on scene were kept to a minimum. In fact, few open-ended questions were posed to any of the interviewees. The interviews were conducted from a script of questions developed by the chief of SIS and were read to each interviewee as if it were merely a formal process in which those being interviewed were there to confirm the chief's preconceived notions of what took place on the scene. The excerpts below are provided verbatim from the written transcripts of the investigations, revealing the leading nature of the questions.

The off-duty lieutenant from Station 2 who had initially reported heavy explosives in the building was asked about my behavior:

Investigator: Okay, was she argumentative or was she just stating the facts?

Lt: No, she was argumentative with the Chief.

Investigator: Okay, was she disrespectful or anything like that?

Lt: Ahm, she was just puttin' her poin—her opinion across that she felt that it was a defensive operation.

The interview with my district chief shows the narrow questions SIS asked:

Investigator: Okay, did she ever indicate during that meeting that she did not trust the qualifications or the judgment of any of the Chief Officers on the fire department? . . .

Investigator: What is your impression of what she was meaning? [Pause] I mean did you read anything into what she was saying, or did you think that she was just second guessing the Chief

> Officers on the scene and that she believed that they had made a bad decision by having crews inside the building?

The written transcripts of each interview were provided to me following the investigation, and it was during my appeals process that I read them in their entirety, only to find that not a single individual on the scene had provided any information that would have indicated the scene was unsafe, the building was becoming unstable, or that my insistence on returning to a defensive attack was appropriate and duly followed.

Following the incident, I had discussed the scene with the lieutenant on Engine 3, the company that had been sent into the structure without a backup line in place. He had stated, "I never wanted to get out of a building as much as that one." He said the stairwell on which they were expected to ascend was crumbling and that there was no way they could have made any progress against the heavy fire on the second floor using only the small-diameter hose with which they had entered. During the interview, he told a different story.

> **Investigator:** Okay. At any time, did the conditions in quadrant A & B deteriorate where it was unsafe?
> **Lt:** No, they did not.

However, four questions later, the lieutenant makes the statement:

> As we worked our way around to the—to the—to a stairwell, that led to the second floor, ah Lt. Bishop (who was there with me) pointed out that he did not feel that the stairwell was safe; due to the fact of its—its charred condition and its lightweight structure.

When Lieutenant Bishop was asked about any safety concerns, he simply replied, "No."

What the investigator and everyone else on scene failed or refused to note was per SOPs, interior crews are not to enter a commercial structure without a backup line in place, meaning that two crews and hose lines enter in unison; crews are never sent in with the understanding that a backup line will eventually follow. The fact that District 2 sent in the crew from Engine 3 before my crew was even assigned to back them up was never brought up.

The tactics on scene were never discussed or questioned. No attention was given to conditions on the fire ground. The appropriateness of my actions was never questioned. Command was never asked whether my actions were justified. The tower crews were never asked about the deteriorating conditions of the building. It seemed no one wanted to acknowledge the tactics or conditions that led to the altercation. It just didn't seem important.

Once the interviews were completed, a meeting was set to present the verdict. It was to take place on duty, at City Hall in the deputy chief's office. There I would be given the verdict of my charges and the subsequent disciplinary action. But during the days leading up to the meeting, another meeting was held between my division chief and a select number of district chiefs in order to determine my punishment. This was highly irregular and completely inappropriate. In fact, I had never heard of such a procedure in my entire career on the department. Disciplinary actions were always handled by the deputy chief of the department. They were never a matter of consensus.

Discipline is usually handed down during a private meeting involving the accused, the deputy chief, and a union representative. The rep is there to ensure that the individual's rights are not violated, which includes adhering to a private format for disciplinary actions (as stated in the Firefighter's Bill of Rights). But my discipline was being decided by a group, many of whom I didn't even work with. The meticulous construction of my punishment would come to light when it was handed down to me.

The day of the meeting arrived and I struggled to calm myself. When it was time to report to City Hall, I walked the short distance from Station 1 and took the elevator up to the seventh floor to Fire Administration. When I arrived, I was told that the meeting would be held in the fire chief's office instead of the deputy chief's. I didn't ask why; I merely followed my district chief down the hall and into the office. When I arrived, the room was crowded with personnel: chiefs, members of SIS, my chain of command, and secretaries from Administration were all crowded around a small table.

I took a seat at the table. The deputy chief then began the meeting. He stated that the investigation had been completed and that today I would be presented with the disciplinary actions decided on by Administration. I thought I would be given time off, in which case I could have opted to use vacation time in its place. I thought perhaps I might be given time off without pay if they really wanted to make a statement. Under the worst-case scenario, I thought I might be removed from the district chief's promotional list. Being removed from the list would have been devastating, not to mention humiliating, but I thought if it happened, I could always retake the test in two years, confident I would score high on the list again and be promoted soon after.

But as the deputy chief handed me the paperwork and announced that I was found guilty on all three charges, he paused before informing me of my punishment. He then made the announcement that would change my career. I was to be removed from the promotional list, stripped of my rank of lieutenant, and demoted to the rank of probationary engineer.

I couldn't speak. I stared at the paperwork in my hand, not comprehending what he was saying. For a split second, I thought perhaps it was all a joke and that they would laugh it off and then discuss the allegations.

But when I looked up, everyone was staring at me, waiting for my response. The first thing I asked him was whether he had read the radio transcripts, which documented the reports of hazardous materials and explosives in the building, the progression of structural weakening, and the fact that District 2 had clearly followed my recommendation on scene to return to a defensive attack after receiving the reports from interior crews.

The chief of the department looked at me and said, "It doesn't matter whether you were right or wrong, we don't argue orders on fire scenes." I didn't even know how to respond to such a ridiculous statement. Of course it mattered whether I was right or wrong. If I had been making some erroneous argument to a chief on scene, with no justification for my actions, it would clearly be a case of inappropriate actions by a subordinate. But I knew the interior crews would meet with heavy fire on the second floor, having seen it from the front of the structure, and I also knew that the building itself had been heavily impacted from the burning of oil and other hazardous fluids; I had seen it with my own two eyes while fighting the fire from Side 1. I also knew that a single engine company with a 1¾" hand line would be no match against a warehouse full of flammable liquids and that Engine 3's crew would be forced to turn back. That is why I had urged District 2 to ask for a radio report. As soon as he did, he ordered them to evacuate. I knew that any administrator should weigh a person's actions against the appropriateness of those actions, and I felt mine had been justified, considering the events on scene.

I asked the chief how he could discount the events surrounding the altercation, especially considering the fact that District 2 had taken my advice and pulled the crews out. But he was unmoved and had little else to say.

They told me I could return to Station 1, pack up my gear, and take the rest of the shift off. I would be informed of my new station assignment within a few days. I was led out of the room by my union representative, who had said nothing during the meeting and seemed to have little to add. I went into the ladies room, trying to pull myself together, placing wet paper towels over my eyes. As furious as I was, I couldn't stop crying, which only added to my aggravation. I hated that all those people had seen me break down, that I had been demoted in front of a crowd of individuals that had no right to be there, as if it were some spectator sport. I could almost hear the phone calls streaming out of City Hall, describing the meeting and spreading the news.

Looking back on this moment, over ten years out, I hate myself for my weakness. I should have stood up, told them all to go fuck themselves, torn up my paperwork, and left. There was nothing else they could do to me. Everything had been taken: my rank, my respect, my dignity, my strength. I hate the fact that I passively accepted the demotion without a fight, without turning my back on all of them and walking away from the department forever.

I joined Mark, my union rep in one of the side offices. I didn't know what to say or how to act. He said very little. The chief entered the office, speaking in subdued tones, trying to keep me calm. He said, "This is just a little blip in your career. You can recover and retake the promotional tests." I stared at him in disbelief. Being demoted was no blip; it was devastating to my reputation and would stick with me my entire career. Not only was I demoted, but having been demoted to a "probationary" status meant I wouldn't be eligible to take the next lieutenant's exam, which was scheduled for the following spring. By making me probationary, they had guaranteed that I would remain in the rank of engineer for the next three years. I realized immediately that this clever means of keeping my career in a standstill for the next few years had been the result of the chiefs' meeting the previous week.

Gone was all I had worked for: my rank of lieutenant, scoring third on the district chief's exam, and all the work it had taken to get to that point. I thought about all the tactical courses I had attended in preparation of becoming a district chief. It was all gone in a matter of moments. Those few minutes on scene—my urgent pleas for a change in tactics—had meant the end of all I had worked for, along with the reputation I had spent a career building. On the day I was demoted, I was two weeks from being promoted to district chief.

AFTERMATH

Companies may have the desire to lay hose and put water on the fire utilizing the fastest, shortest, most direct route. This process is called the "candle moth" syndrome and may draw a company to attack a fire from the burned side, which should be avoided.

—OFD OFFENSIVE OPERATIONS

MARK AND I WALKED BACK TO STATION 1, SAYING LITTLE ON THE way. Mark and I had been friends for a long time. I knew he was concerned, but could find few words. I still couldn't get my mind around the fact that I was no longer a lieutenant. The implications set in quickly. I would have to turn in my white officer's shirts and return to wearing the blue shirts I had left behind once I made rank. I would have to turn in my red officer's helmet and return to my battered leather I had used for so many years. Where would I be stationed? How would I ever face members of my department? My mind raced through the humiliation of it all.

Mark reminded me it was just a job, not to do anything "rash." I assured him I would never harm myself over this, that the job wasn't worth my life. The whole discussion struck me as ludicrous. I had fought hard my entire career. I had made it through the death of my mother when I was twenty-three; I knew I would make it through this. I just wasn't sure I wanted to stick around to see it through.

When we arrived back at Station 1, I gathered my gear and fled. I couldn't face anyone. I just wanted to escape and try to get my head together. As I got in my car, a thought flashed in my mind: how was I ever going to tell my father?

As a career naval officer, my father understood the challenges and significance of rank. He had been so proud of my promotion to lieutenant and excited at the prospect of my pending promotion as only the second female in the history of the department to achieve the rank of district chief.

I stopped at my apartment to change out of my uniform, wondering if it would be the last time I ever wore the white shirt of an officer. I drove to his home and went inside. He knew I had been anxious about the pending investigation and had been supportive, believing it would blow over and I would get through it. I entered his living room to find him and my stepmother enjoying a quiet afternoon. I tried to keep it together as I told him about the events of the day. I described the meeting and then broke down as I told him about the demotion. He simply looked at me, stunned into silence. I told him I felt I had no options, that my reputation was ruined and that I had to resign. On the drive over, I had started to assess my options.

It was September. Had I accepted the position within the graduate program at Florida State University, I would have just been starting coursework. Perhaps it wasn't too late. I could write to the anthropology department and explain that my situation had changed, that I would be coming after all.

My father listened patiently, telling me that I had to follow my instincts. Having spent his life in the military, he was well-versed in the machinations of rank and the consequences of demotion. He let me vent my rage and frustration at the department, its total disregard for my intentions on scene and the work and dedication that had gone into my career. He asked if there was an appeals process. I assured him the union would take up the matter and that my case should be forwarded for a formal appeal in front of an arbitrator. He urged me to pursue all options within the department before leaving behind all I had worked for. I assured him I would work with the union to see that the arbitration went forward and that I would also pursue an interdepartmental appeal, which was granted in serious cases.

I left his house and returned home. The next few days passed in a blur. I was visited by Mark and our union president, Steve, who informed me I would remain on C Shift but would be assigned to Station 11. I was appalled. Station 11 was known as the good old boys' station, filled with backslapping guys who loved to sit around and talk about hunting. I could think of no worse place for someone in my position. I knew they would make life hard for me. I asked if there was any possibility I could remain at Station 1. That way, I would at least be among people I knew and was used to working with. But the union men assured me the assignment would not be changed.

Mark told me I could take as much time off as needed before reporting to Station 11. I told him I would rather get it over with—time wasn't going to change the fact that I was to return to shift as a probationary engineer. The probationary designation meant I was forced to work under the supervision of a lieutenant and that I had lost the privilege of "riding out of grade." Although I had been working as a lieutenant and riding out of grade as a district chief in preparation for my promotion, I was now restricted to driving a truck. I told them I would report to duty in a few days.

The next day, I took my white shirts and red helmet to Supply, where we obtained our uniforms and gear. I parked behind the building, hoping not to run into anyone as I carried the clothing and gear of my past rank inside. Ed, the supply officer with whom I had worked for many years, met me at the door, giving me a big hug as I handed him the helmet and shirts. I left quickly and returned home, where I holed up throughout the weekend, planning my return to shift.

I would report to duty and not discuss the case. I would stay quiet, perform my duties as an engineer, and never let those bastards see that I was crushed. I would stay strong and focused. I would plan to appeal the case and attend the next union meeting, where I would ask for backing in sending the case to arbitration. I had to think; I had to plan. After the initial shock, I began my strategy.

Under the best-case scenario, I would appeal internally and go before a panel of departmental officers to plead my case. Should the internal appeals not work, I would go before the union and ask for arbitration. In cases such as this, the union would set up arbitration to allow a member to go before a board made up of officers from other departments, in order to ensure an unbiased review. Perhaps one of these processes would reverse the demotion. If I could only get my rank back, I knew I could work through the controversy. Although I knew my reputation would be forever stained by the event, I would not let other's opinions impact my ability and desire to serve as an officer.

The weekend slipped away and I prepared for duty at Station 11. It would be even worse that I imagined.

REPORTING FOR DUTY

The effect of the interior attack must be evaluated and the attack abandoned if necessary.

—OFD OFFENSIVE OPERATIONS

I'LL NEVER FORGET WALKING INTO STATION 11 ON THE FIRST DAY OF my demoted status. Just being back in a blue shirt was embarrassing enough, a blatant reminder of my lack of rank. I put my gear on the truck and started my checkout. I knew the guys at Station 11, having worked there years before as a firefighter. They were a rowdy bunch who loved to play practical jokes and sit around the kitchen telling stories of their hunting adventures. I had always felt out of place there; the fact that I had gone from a district chief candidate to a probationary engineer made it even more uncomfortable, and I heard their whispers as I was unloading my gear.

As I finished my truck checkout, a couple of them came out into the bay, advising me that the mops and brooms were in the side closet. They found it hilarious that I was now forced to clean the station as one of them.

I kept to myself. I stayed in one of the back offices, reading most of the day. My new district chief soon informed me that as a probationary engineer, I would be forced to take a "street test" for Station 11's territory. Each new probationary engineer is required to take a test to ensure they know the location of each street, hydrant, and major building in their area. It was humiliating to be made to take it again, since I had already passed that hurdle when I had originally been promoted to engineer. It was simply another means of embarrassing me and highlighting my status as driver. So I started studying the streets within the area, my frustration growing with each shift.

The guys would make jibes at me whenever they could. When I received phone calls, they would not simply say "Smith, Line 1" (Smith being my maiden name). They would always say "Engineer Smith" to remind me of my lowly status. On weekends, they would check out their trucks and then settle into the kitchen for a long breakfast. Saturdays were designated as "station cleanup." Since I didn't enjoy huge breakfasts and had no desire to sit around discussing departmental gossip with them, I would complete my checkout and get started on my share of the cleanup.

One Saturday, a week or so into my demotion, I started morning cleanup as they enjoyed their breakfast and chatter. I swept and mopped, cleaning up the puddles of black grease that seem to perpetually drip from the trucks. I knocked down cobwebs and straightened equipment. There was little left to do so I hid out in the back office, reading as usual. I figured the other two engineers would take care of the few chores left within the bay.

But after a while, I was called over the loudspeaker. "Engineer Smith, report to the bay for cleanup." I was furious. I had already done the majority of the chores and wanted to be left alone. But the other engineers reminded me that chores were done "as a crew," and that we would all work together until they were completed. The fact that they had been sitting on their asses the entire time I worked made no difference to them. This was simply an opportunity for them to order me to perform cleanup. I appealed to the lieutenant, who merely shrugged and advised me to "just keep your head down."

As the shifts wore on, I became more embittered. It was infuriating to have guys on the department with half my seniority now ordering me around and getting pleasure from my humiliation. And the harassment wasn't limited to my station personnel.

One afternoon, I was sitting in the darkened living room of the station. It had been a busy shift and I was tired and sweaty. I felt worn out and even thought about going home sick, something I rarely did. Each shift was a reminder of my lowly status. I had lost all camaraderie with the guys on the department. It felt as if they all looked upon me with ridicule and condescension. My job was no longer a source of pride and enjoyment; it was a daily reminder of my failures.

The phone rang and my name was called over the intercom: "Engineer Smith, line 1." I picked up the phone and was met by an angry voice at the other end.

"You were a lousy lieutenant and you got what you deserved."

I sat there, thinking that if this was one of my friends, it was a lousy joke. But it was no joke. Someone—an older male from what I could tell by the voice on the phone—was actually calling me anonymously to ridicule me over the phone. I slammed the phone down, unable to believe that somewhere, someone on the department was hateful enough to make a crank call. I sat there, stunned, unable to believe it yet unable to get the voice out of my head. I reported it to the lieutenant and SIS was notified, but nothing was done. What could be done for such a juvenile act?

Along with my frustration, I had become incredibly paranoid on duty. What if I wrecked the truck? What if I gave a wrong dose of meds to a patient? I had lost faith in my own abilities and was scared of making another mistake. I no longer trusted my own judgment. I thought I had been doing my duty when I confronted District 2. What if I could no longer trust my intuition? In an emergency, if you couldn't trust your gut, you were in big trouble. I couldn't sleep at night on duty. It was like my nerves were constantly coiled and my actions under a microscope.

I knew my case was still the hot gossip around the department. I caught wind of stories people were spreading describing my actions on scene. One of the guys even confronted me one day in the kitchen about the incident, demanding me to justify my actions in front of everyone. I had worked with Pat before and knew he could be a bullying asshole. I had seen him harass other guys on the department, goading them until they stormed out of the room in frustration. I tried to explain what had actually happened on scene, but he just waived his hand in front of my face, dismissing my explanation and laughing as the other guys stood uncomfortably by.

I finally realized my explanations were useless. He and everyone else would believe what they wanted to believe about the incident. By this point the incident had been gossip fodder among the department for several weeks. Everyone had made up their minds as to who was at fault. To them, my demotion was simply confirmation of my guilt.

THE APPEAL

A simple rule to follow would be: "big fire" use "big water." While a 1¾ inch attack line offers mobility, it is ineffective in commercial fires with a large load.

—OFD COMMERCIAL BUILDING OPERATIONS

I BECAME MORE SECLUDED ON DUTY, NOT WANTING TO INTERACT with the crews. I received word from administration that my appeal would be heard and a date was set to go before select members of fire administration to plead my case. I was approached by Kathy, the lone female who had broken through to achieve the rank of district chief, who offered to help with my appeal. We spent the next couple of weeks pouring over the radio transmissions, reviewing the layout of the building, and highlighting provisions within the SOPs that require an officer to pass on information critical to the safety of fire-ground operations.

We also focused on the discrepancies in tactics on the scene. It is always easy to criticize the actions on scene following an emergency incident. As an incident unfolds, you deal with the information you have on hand. Things seem much clearer in hindsight, when full details have been revealed and the incident is over. In the midst of the incident, without all the information at hand, one is guided by judgment and tactical knowledge. We all do the best we can.

But there were obvious tactical flaws made during the incident. I came to realize it was these flaws that no one wanted to address and, to make matters worse, I was being perceived as disloyal for raising them now.

Considering the information that was provided to first-arriving crews at the fire—primarily the heavy loads of hazardous materials, the presence of heavy explosives in the building, and the fact that all employees had been evacuated—the fire should have been deemed a "surround and drown" situation, since there were numerous hazards yet no life safety issues (no civilians to rescue). Just because the initial fire had been knocked down did not change the reports of explosives and hazardous materials within the building. The intensity of fire within the structure was not only compounded by the building's contents; the building itself was becoming unstable, as reported by the tower crews who noted cracks and sags in the sides and roof of the structure.

Another major breach in tactics was sending Engine 3 in without a backup line and with nothing but a small-diameter hand line. We had been fighting the fire from the front of the building with two large-diameter hoses and still could not completely extinguish the fire. The fact that District 2 had sent Engine 3 in without backup in place and with a small hand line was something he should have had to answer for, a total breach in fire tactics involving large commercial structures. There would be no way he could justify it. His radio reports make it clear he was concerned that Engine 3 was inside without a backup. Yet he had sent them in several minutes prior to backup crews even being assigned to his location.

Finally, I hoped that the fact that District 2 had followed my urging to pull out interior crews would validate my actions on scene. My arguments had clearly been on point, since the entire scenario shifted to a defensive mode following my urging. I felt sure the appeals board would see the hypocrisy in charging me with insubordination, failure to obey, and failure to assist when, had it not been for my insistence, he may have kept the crews inside as the building crumbled around them.

But when I learned of the makeup of the appeals board, my heart sank. The board would be headed by a division chief I had worked with for many years. Although we were on good terms and had always got along, Dave was notoriously sexist and would constantly make embarrassing comments to me in front of my crew members. He would saunter into the station, loudly making jokes and calling attention to himself, and would always approach me with the same remark: "Why don't you go put on some more makeup!"

This always got a laugh out of the guys, since he was popular among the men. But this remark and many others he made were humiliating and inappropriate, especially coming from a chief. Many times I would not make eye contact with him when he entered, hoping to avoid his attention. I don't believe he intended to be hurtful, but he had no clue as to the effect his words had on those on the receiving end. Dave loved being the center of attention around the stations and I knew he found great pleasure in humiliating those around him. My hopes for a fair appeal quickly faded.

The other member of the board was a serious-minded division chief who had his eye on becoming chief of the department. His ambitions were notorious and he was constantly posturing for upper administration. But his solemnity gave me hope. He took his responsibilities seriously and I hoped he would balance what I knew would be Dave's reckless approach to the case. Although a competent fire officer, Dave approached most aspects of the department with an attitude of ridicule and disrespect. I couldn't imagine how he had been selected to lead an appeals process of such a serious nature unless Administration simply wasn't taking it seriously.

Kathy and I worked to prepare my case. To this day, I don't know if her support helped or hurt me. She was greatly supportive and was a good tactician. She was smart and methodical in laying out my case. But she had struggled within the department her entire career. As the first female to achieve rank, she had been butting her head against the glass ceiling for so long that she tended to come across as guarded and defensive. Her assistance was greatly appreciated, but I felt we were seen as just two more females trying to break into what should remain a "guy's realm."

The day of the appeal arrived and we met early to lay out our materials. We had photos of the scene, taken in the early stages of the fire to show its intensity as units arrived on scene. We had a timeline of the radio transmissions and the applicable SOPs highlighted to show that I was following the departmental guidelines in confronting District 2's orders for the interior attack. Both chiefs listened, the serious one studying the radio transmissions, Dave leaning back in his chair, occasionally glancing at the ceiling.

They questioned my actions on scene and it was the first opportunity I had to thoroughly explain what I had seen, what I had felt on arriving at the rear of the structure to see interior hose lines, and the urgency I had felt about having interior crews removed. At one point, I said that I knew Engine 3 was going to encounter heavy fire on the second floor, having seen it from the front of the building. The serious chief looked at me and said sarcastically, "That's their job!" He seemed unconcerned about the reports concerning the building's hazardous contents or its failing integrity. Nothing I said moved him.

At the end of our presentation, they asked if I had anything else to add. I had prepared a statement that I tried to read without breaking down. It recounted my history with the department, my educational achievements, my work as an administrative lieutenant within the Training Department, and the hard work it had taken to achieve my rank. I knew that my options were dwindling and that if this appeal did not overturn the demotion, I had only arbitration left. I struggled through the statement, at one point being interrupted by Dave, who casually asked if I wanted to "go get myself together before continuing." I shook my head and finished the statement, once again ashamed and frustrated that I had broken down in front of them.

They dismissed me and said I would be informed of their decision. Within twenty-four hours they notified me that they had no intention of reversing the charges or the disciplinary action. The union would be my only hope.

TURNING TO THE UNION

Command cannot lose sight of the very simple and basic fireground reality that at some point the fire forces must engage the fire and fight.

—OFD OFFENSIVE OPERATIONS

THE INTERNATIONAL ASSOCIATION OF FIRE FIGHTERS (IAFF) LOCAL 1365, the collective bargaining unit for OFD, is one of the strongest unions in Florida. Chartered in 1960, it has grown in strength and influence throughout its history and is a force to be reckoned with when it comes to contract negotiations. Well connected politically, the union is primarily responsible for the lucrative contracts and benefits enjoyed by members of OFD. It is also tasked with protecting personnel charged with rules or conduct violations.

The union has a long history of fighting for members. Even nonmembers are provided protection and backing when charged with a violation. During my tenure with OFD, the union had backed personnel during investigations for minor offenses, such as excessive incidents of reporting late for duty; it had supported several members charged with DUI, negotiating terms for their continued employment; and it had even stood behind members charged with drug violations. I can recall no instance when the union refused to back a member of the department. I had been a union member since joining the department and expected full support. I would be sorely mistaken.

Once the internal appeal was completed, I met with Steve, the union president, to discuss arbitration. I had known Steve for many years. He was well connected and influential among the members of the department. I believed at the beginning of the case that Steve could have quashed much of the gossip circulating within the department. I had hoped he would quell the bashing my reputation was taking, reminding members that I had a clean work history and had worked hard for my achievements. But none of that happened. He seemed to be carried along with the gossip, even enjoining the drama of it all and the upcoming role the union would play in my defense. He said arbitration would depend on a vote from the union board. I was worried.

For the majority of my career with OFD, our union board was made up of seasoned veterans, many of them lieutenants, who had spent years on the department as it grew in size and reputation. For many years, the president was a thoughtful, soft-spoken lieutenant known for his careful words and meticulous approach to problems. But the union had been through many changes in the late 1990s. Steve was voted in as president when the former president decided to step down pending his retirement. The board was replaced by several young members, many with only a few years on the department who had not yet achieved rank. Although rank was not a requirement for the positions on the board, those who had been through promotional processes and held supervisory positions on the department typically had better perspectives on matters concerning administration and politics. Once the new board took over, the tenor of the union changed to a more short-sighted, less disciplined organization. Gone was the thoughtful, calculated approach to departmental matters. This new union chose petty battles with administration, bragging when it prevailed, trash-talking when it didn't.

Fire Administration had changed as well. The union had fought to remove the previous fire chief, a man who had presided over another large department in Florida and who had a reputation for strict professionalism and structure. This approach was new to OFD. The previous chief had been a member of the department his entire career. He was a strong, decisive leader and well liked among the members. He maintained a cozy relationship with the union, conducting much of their negotiations behind closed doors or over beers.

When the new chief took office, ushering in a more formal approach to administration, the union was dismayed to find that the open-door policies of the former administration were no longer in place and that the union had to conduct negotiations as the chief saw fit, not on its whim. He didn't last long. The mayor's race was approaching and she relied on heavy support from the union. The union made it clear that she would have that support in exchange for the replacement of the chief. He was gone in a matter of months. The mayor went on to be reelected.

The new board made me nervous. I knew many of them, some better than others. I was worried about maintaining their support, knowing the heated gossip that continued to circulate throughout the department. Even after my demotion, the case was still the topic of conversation, everyone wondering about the pending arbitration process, knowing a vote would decide my fate. My only option at this point was to go before an arbitrator and argue my case. I felt confident that if I could get someone to review the tactics on scene, my actions would be justified and I could be reinstated as a lieutenant. If only they would look at the tactics . . .

The board could vote no. If it decided not to support me, I could opt to pay for the arbitration myself, which was around $3,000. But the thought of going to arbitration on my own made me furious. I was a union member and expected union support. The union owed me the protection that comes with membership, and I was not willing to let the board off the hook and pursue arbitration myself. If the board voted me down, that would be the last straw and I would leave the department. The vote would be the deciding factor.

As I wrapped up my meeting with Steve, I asked him, "What would you have done in my position on scene?"

He thought for a moment before responding, "I would have gone in."

"Even with what I had seen from Side 1, the reports of hazardous materials and explosives, and the lack of communication concerning the change in tactics?" I said, astounded.

"Even so," he said. "I would have entered the building then radioed command that we couldn't make forward progress."

"So you would have bullshitted your way out?" I asked.

"Yes," he replied.

"I guess I was at fault for thinking I could be honest and rely on good judgment," I said.

THE MEETING

Determine fire location and extent before starting fire operations (as far as possible). Avoid operating fire streams into smoke.

—OFD OFFENSIVE OPERATIONS

UNION MEETINGS ALWAYS FELL ON A TUESDAY NIGHT. MY CASE WAS put on the agenda and I waited apprehensively as the date approached. In the meantime, I sent out an email to my friends and those I had worked with in the past, asking for their support. I received few responses. Dan, a friend I had known my entire career, was one of the few who wrote back. His response shocked me. He said that although we had been friends for many years, he felt in his heart he could not support me after hearing how I had behaved on scene. I hadn't spoken to Dan since the incident, so I knew he was getting his information via the gossip around the department. I called him the next morning when I got off shift.

He was nervous when he heard my voice on the receiver. I could tell he didn't want to discuss the matter, but he stayed on the phone and listened quietly as I took him through the incident. When I finished, he was silent for several seconds. When he finally spoke, he confirmed my worst fears.

He said my account of the incident was completely different from what was being said around the department. He said everyone was discussing how I had screamed at District 2, refusing to enter the building. I told him I never refused the order, which explained why they hadn't charged me with "refusal to obey." Even District 2, if asked, would have to admit I never refused the order. I had only argued for a change in tactics.

Dan was appalled. He couldn't believe how the story had morphed over the past weeks. We discussed the tactics of the fire and again he was amazed that no one was addressing the issues of safety and judgment concerning the decision for an interior attack. I got the same response when explaining my actions to those few members in the department who dared discuss it with me. The story around the department had become so overblown that no one was surprised I had been demoted. The firefighters felt it was a deserved punishment and felt no need to pursue the case. I was worried the union board would feel the same.

The procedure for the vote was a structured process. I would be given time to make a statement, then members would have the opportunity to get up and speak either against me or on my behalf. The rules stated that a vote of arbitration from the board could only be made if three members spoke on my behalf. All I needed was three.

The meeting began and once the opening procedures were completed, my case was brought up for discussion. I sat in the audience, hands shaking as I clutched my statement. I knew it was my only chance to lay out the facts of the case, dispel the rumors that had been circulating, and show that I never refused an order, as so many on the department were saying. I wanted the members to think about the tactics involved, to question their appropriateness in order to understand my actions on scene. I was called to the front of the room where I laid out my statement on the podium and began to speak.

I kept the statement brief. I wanted to present a clear, concise argument. I faced a mixture of stern looks and blank expressions. Many had no intention of speaking; they merely came to observe. The room was packed and as I scanned the crowd, I could see District 2 sitting in the back of the room. Chiefs were not union members at the time. They had no representation and were not supposed to attend union meetings, since issues concerning administration were usually discussed. This policy ensured an open forum for personnel, where they could speak their minds and discuss issues they faced within the department.

But no one on the board questioned his presence or asked him to leave, as they should have. I was forced to make my statement with him staring angrily at me, as if daring to defy him in public.

After laying out the events on scene, I closed my statement by affirming that my concern had been for the safety of interior crews, my purpose for the altercation was to have them removed from interior operations immediately, and that it was my duty as a lieutenant to advise District 2 of what I had seen from Side 1 of the building. I described how District 2 had followed my urgings for a radio report from Engine 3 and that when it was received he immediately removed the crew from interior operations. I assured them I would never disobey a direct order that adhered to the safety provisions within our SOPs and that I had not done so on this scene. I urged the members to ask District 2 himself if I had disobeyed an order. I looked directly at him as I said this, challenging him to speak up, knowing he could not argue the point. He remained silent throughout my statement. I closed by reminding them that any one of them could one day find themselves in my place, needing the backing of the union to obtain arbitration, and as a union member, arbitration was my right .

I returned to my seat and waited for the next phase to begin. All I could hope for was that three members would stand up quickly on my behalf and proclaim that as a union member, I should be afforded the same protection as any other member and that, in spite of personal feelings toward the case or my actions on scene, the union should support my request for arbitration so that I would be assured a fair and unbiased assessment of the case.

This was not to happen quickly. Those that jumped to the front of the line to make a statement were those wanting to grandstand in front of the members. They got up and proclaimed that they were "appalled" at someone who would "abandon their brothers in their time of need." One by one, they stood in front of the crowded room and proclaimed me a coward, one that didn't deserve the backing of the union.

In my mind I was screaming, *"You motherfuckers! I've worked my ass off on this department, fighting fires next to many of you for eleven years! Do you think I just woke up that morning and decided I didn't want to enter a burning building?!"*

Their statements went on for about twenty minutes. I stood in the back of the room, too anxious to remain seated and not wanting to have others staring at me as the brutal accusations were made. Since the board members sat at the front of the room, I wanted to make each of them look at me when casting their vote. They sat in silence, many of the men rifling through paperwork on the table before them, insensible to the proceedings that were deciding my fate. Finally, as the most vocal of the members finished their statements, slapping each other on the back as they returned to their seats, proud of their bold assertions against me, members in support of me began to speak up.

Their arguments were more tempered than the ones against me. One of my former partners stated that arbitration is a right of all members and that in spite of personal feelings, I deserved the chance for the case to be reviewed. I appreciated his thoughtful statement and hoped it would sway the board.

I hoped the board would keep in mind the purpose behind arbitration. It provided a fair and unbiased review of the case, one removed from the influence of politics within the department. I knew this was the key to my success—to get fire officers from outside of the department to review the tactics on scene and take them into consideration when judging my actions, since neither the investigation nor the internal review had included an assessment of the tactics in their evaluation of my case. I thought about what the chief had said at my demotion, *"It doesn't matter if you were right or wrong; we don't disobey orders on fire scenes."* I knew this reasoning wouldn't stand up in an external appeal.

Finally, I had the three required endorsements and the vote was placed before the board. I watched as the majority of hands rose to vote against me. The case would not be sent to arbitration. I could pursue it on my own, at my own expense, should I wish to do so. Otherwise, the board felt the matter was closed. I stood there silently as the board moved on to new business.

I slipped out of the union hall, speaking to no one, and made my way through the dark parking lot to my car. The events of the past few weeks flashed through my mind, a blur of stress, humiliation, and defeat. There was but one final option; it was time for me to leave OFD.

THE ONLY OPTION

Command must develop critical decisions that relate to cut-off points and must approach fire spread determinations with pessimism.

—OFD OFFENSIVE OPERATIONS

I LEFT THE NEXT MORNING TO FLY TO IDAHO TO SPEND THANKSGIVING with my brother. It was a great escape, getting on the plane, knowing I was traveling far from all that had plagued me over the last few weeks. I looked forward to discussing my plans with my brother. I needed to map out the next few weeks and knew he would provide support and encouragement

We spent several days, huddled inside against the snow and wind of Idaho's approaching winter, sipping gin and talking. I discussed the case, replaying the events of the last month in all their frustrating detail. I told him I felt there was no alternative at this point but to leave the department and pursue grad school. I knew my reputation on the department was forever impacted, that it would take years to rebuild all that I had achieved at the time of the demotion. I had no intention of repeating the struggles of the last five years and could not fathom working under the supervision of a lieutenant after serving in that rank for two years. I also felt that to stay at OFD would be a waste of my education and experience.

As the events of the case had unfolded, after each failed attempt at retribution, my loyalty to the department and my dedication as a firefighter had slowly been torn down. I no longer felt a part of the department. I felt like an outsider, forever relegated to a shameful position among my peers. My confidence on the job was gone; the cocky firefighter I had once been was replaced by a disillusioned individual who would forever carry a chip on her shoulder. No matter what achievements I made in the future, no matter how many additional promotional tests I took, I would never recapture the trust and respect I once held as an officer on the department.

But my future was not lost. All the years I had spent getting educated would finally pay off. One of the motivations for achieving a bachelor's and master's degree was to ensure that I would have options, should I decide one day to end my career in the fire service. All those times I studied as the guys made fun of my educational pursuits, teasing me for reading "books about bones" and "that science crap," would enable me to move on to other fields, should I ever decide to do so. Another benefit to my years on the department was that after ten years of service I had become vested in my pension. I wouldn't be resigning; I would be retiring with eleven years of service and would receive a pension when I turned forty-seven.

My father had always told me, "Educational achievement is the one thing no one can ever take from you." He was right. They could strip me of my rank, they could tear down my reputation, and they could destroy all that I had built, but they couldn't change the fact that I was a woman with multiple degrees and years of experience under my belt. My career as a firefighter might be over, but the next phase was just beginning.

As the holiday weekend came to a close and I landed in Salt Lake City to make the connecting flight back to Orlando, I called FSU's Admissions Department to have the necessary paperwork forwarded so that I could join the graduate program in January. I had called the chair of anthropology, Dr. Glen Doran, to discuss the possibility of reactivating my acceptance into the department. He assured me that since I had been accepted for the fall semester, it would be highly likely I would be accepted again if I were to enter the program as a post-baccalaureate student. I could enter classes in January and apply after I arrived. Although the thought of giving up my life in Orlando without a definite guarantee of admission made me nervous, I was willing to gamble. I made the reactivation deadline by one day.

I had drafted my letter of retirement early one morning before leaving Idaho. It was a cold morning and a light snow was falling. I had slept little, going over the wording of the letter in my head throughout the long night. It felt good to put it down on paper, a final severing of my ties with the department. My retirement date would be January 1, 2001. I had enough accumulated sick leave to take me through the month of December, so I requested to "burn" it. I was never going to report to shift again. It was hard to accept the fact that I would never again step foot on a fire truck, but I refused to return to the humiliation of working as an engineer.

I took the letter to City Hall, leaving it on the chief's desk for him to find when he returned to his office. I received a phone call from him later that day, requesting me to come to his office the next morning to discuss my retirement. I arrived in his office and we sat down to talk. He urged me to reconsider. He said he recognized the fact that I had worked hard throughout my career and was confident I could reclaim my status as a lieutenant in a few short years. I told him it didn't matter if I retook the exam—I would never be able to live down the events surrounding the case. And most of all, my heart was no longer in it.

I felt I had given everything I had to the department. I had worked hard, studied hard, and performed to the best of my abilities. But it wasn't enough. I told him I felt the investigation of the case had been a joke. There never should have been an investigation. I told him we both knew that emergency scenes are often chaotic and that officers relied on each other for information and input. My actions on scene were driven by a sense of urgency for those inside the building. I felt the tactics on scene had been reckless and that I was being made to suffer for standing up to a district chief who appeared untouchable and free from responsibility.

District 2's actions should have been reviewed. The entire scenario should have been considered, not dismissed as if it were unconnected to my actions on scene. That the department would demote me without placing my actions in context proved to me that OFD had no intention of actually determining if I was wrong or right; the investigation merely served as an outlet for District 2's anger over being challenged on scene. I finished by saying that if OFD was a department that relied on officers who blindly followed orders, then I no longer had any interest in working there. I assured him I would not change my mind and thanked him for his time. I left his office for the last time.

The chief granted my request to burn my sick leave. I went by Station 11 early one morning on an off-shift, not wanting to see any of my former crew. I gathered my belongings, loading them into my car for the final time. I went by Supply and turned in my gear. I would never again feel the weight of an air pack on my back; I would never feel the security of my bunker gear; I would never feel the rush of air hitting my face as I strapped on my mask. The familiarities of over a decade of firefighting would be part of my past. The camaraderie I once loved had faded into the past. It was time to look forward, to plan the days, months, and years ahead. It was time for a new life.

FAREWELL

Write-off property that is already lost and go on to protect exposed property based on the most dangerous direction of spread. Do not continue to operate in positions that are essentially lost.

—OFD OFFENSIVE OPERATIONS

I IMMEDIATELY PUT MY CONDO ON THE MARKET AND STARTED MAKing arrangements for the move. I went to Tallahassee to find an apartment, staying in a rustic bed and breakfast in the heart of the city's historic downtown. The rich canopied landscape of the city was a welcomed change and I felt nervous and excited, knowing this would be my new home in a matter of weeks. I arrived in town on a rainy Sunday, the sky gray and heavy above my head. I spent the afternoon searching the classified ads for apartments in the area. I mapped out several to look at the next morning and settled into my room as the rain continued.

The future scared me. I was leaving a secure job, with great pay and benefits and a beautiful home that I loved. I was exchanging it for an uncertain future, entering a graduate program with no assurance of success or completion. I was relying on my instincts and motivation to get me through. But I was determined to succeed.

After finding an apartment and filling out the necessary paperwork, I headed back to Orlando to prepare for the move. My condo sold within ten days, a cash deal for just under my asking price—a good omen. We closed the deal within a week and before I knew it, I was packed and heading to FSU.

I settled into my new apartment and began classes within a week. It was strange to be removed from the life I had known for so long, the familiarity of my life in Orlando. The coursework was heavy, which gave me focus and clarity.

But the nights were hard. I was plagued with insomnia. I found myself replaying the events of the last few months over and over again in my head, reliving the shame and humiliation of my demotion. My dreams revolved around the department. They passed as flashes upon my subconscious, scenes of conflict and indignity. I thought living in a new place, with new responsibilities, would enable me to separate myself from the past. But it stayed with me, draping my thoughts in a heavy cloak of mourning.

I mourned the loss of my career. I mourned the wonderful memories from years in the field, those amazing experiences in human emotion. I mourned the loss of the young woman I had been when I entered the field of EMS, knowing those years were forever behind me and that the person of my youth had been transformed by my experiences, for better and worse.

But I found strength in mourning. I remembered what it had been like, days after my mother had died, the emptiness that had settled in my chest, the hollowness that encased my life during those first months. When she was sick, I believed if she died I would die too. I couldn't imagine life beyond her death. Following her death, I was amazed to find that life continued, that I pushed on in spite of the overwhelming sense of loss.

That experience taught me that I could survive anything. I knew that after making it through the loss of my mother, nothing could ever tear me down. The firefighter may have been broken, my career destroyed, but they would never break me as an individual. Her death taught me that through painful events we find inner strength and determination. It was the greatest lesson of my life.

It has been eleven years since I left OFD. I completed my master's degree and went straight into the PhD program, completing my doctoral degree in just three years. I have learned more during this time than I ever thought possible. I have pushed myself well beyond the goals I once set within the fire service, beyond anything I could have imagined as a young girl of twenty-three when I first entered paramedic school.

Those years are irreplaceable. The lessons I learned, the things I saw, the people I worked with, the patients I treated—all of it shaped who I am today. My years as a firefighter and paramedic will forever be the years that ushered me into adulthood. I witnessed life through the children I delivered; I witnessed death in the patients I lost; I stood face-to-face with the destructive force of fire; I felt the warmth and camaraderie of working with those whose lives depend on each other. I feel fortunate to have been a part of all of that.

I think about the string of events leading to my demotion: the altercation on scene; the fury it caused District 2, being challenged on scene by a subordinate; the investigation that should have evaluated the tactics surrounding my challenge; the unprecedented lack of support by the union. Had any of these events turned out differently, the resulting demotion might not have occurred, and today I would be approaching retirement following a long career with OFD. But these events did take place and altered everything in their wake. It shattered a hard-fought career that had seemed so perfect in the making, yet ended so badly.

Perhaps my case was doomed from the start. I was not only going up against District 2; I was going up against a tradition steeped in history. OFD prided itself on its adherence to aggressive interior attacks. By approaching firefighting from any other perspective, even those based on the latest tactics that stressed safety over aggression, I was placing myself outside the playing field, beyond the lines that define the machismo of firefighting.

For me, the hardest part of the incident was that none of my coworkers ever gave me the benefit of the doubt. These were people I had worked closely with for over a decade. I had served to the best of my ability, working hard, educating myself in order to be the best officer I could be. These men knew me; I was one of them. I had worked my way up the ladder and was perched to make it even higher when it all came crashing down. Had it not been for my pending promotion to district chief, I feel confident my discipline would not have been as severe. It was as if the more that was at stake, the more destructive my discipline became.

Was it strictly sexist? No, I don't think anyone set out to crush my career merely because I was a female. But I'm confident it was a contributing factor. I saw how attitudes changed as I worked my way up through the ranks. I felt the change in my coworkers, the shift in acceptance, the diminution of my inclusion as "one of them." I knew going into the field of firefighting that, as a female, I would be relegated to the periphery, that the "brotherhood" would remain an impenetrable realm of the masculine arena of fighting fire. I accepted that early on.

I've spent many years reviewing my decisions on scene. I think back to the morning of the call. I remember the intense heat of that August day, the anticipation of responding to the fire, and the thick column of black smoke on the horizon as we sped through the city, sirens screaming. The scene unfolds in my mind's eye: the noise and confusion as we positioned our truck; red lights flashing through the humid, smoky air; and the order for me to report to the rear of the building to District 2's sector. I remember my shock at seeing a hose line snaking its way into the darkened interior, knowing there were men on the other end heading deep into a building weakened by fire, full of burning flammable liquids. I hear the radio reports of heavy explosives, the recommendation to "go defensive," and the anger in District 2's face when I insist he pull them out.

But the radio transmissions tell the real story. They are an unbiased account of each moment on scene, an archive of the event that ended my career. They reveal what really happened, apart from the gossip and exaggeration that followed. Had they been admitted into the investigation and critiqued along with my actions, there is not a firefighter on the department who would not have understood the concern I felt for the interior crews, the level of danger inherent in the tactics utilized on scene, and the urgency in my confrontation with District 2. He knew he was wrong to send in crews without a backup line in place; he knew he was risking those crews, not to save lives but so that he could be the one to make an aggressive attack on the fire. Three minutes into his interior attack, Command advises him there is fire through the roof, yet he still allows interior crews to continue, ordering my crew to go in as well. Our confrontation over tactics, my urgent pleas to pull them out, and my insistence for a return to defensive operations forced him to confront the fact that his attack was unsuccessful and unnecessary, and he was furious that it was a female subordinate who forced his hand.

That an entire career can be lost in a single moment is still a hard thing for me to accept. But I spent a career seeing lives altered in the split second it takes to fire a gun, crash a car, or stop a heart.

The incidents that led to the end of my career in no way diminish the years of happiness and fulfillment that formed its majority. Although it has taken me over a decade to accept and overcome those last months on the department, I have arrived on the other side of the pain and humiliation of that period. I accept responsibility for my actions and know I was reacting with the safety of the interior crews in mind. Was it worth losing my career over? The only peace I take from the incident is that we all made it back to the station that afternoon.

Each of us is shaped by our experiences. We go through life acting and reacting to the things around us based on how we see the world and the emotional lessons of our past. My reactions on scene were based on my experiences in the field. Had I not had a close call two years before the incident, perhaps I would not have approached the scene with such caution. But had I not been as cautious, perhaps I would not be recounting the events today.

We cannot know the future. We can only plan and react with as much honesty and thoughtfulness with which we are capable. The events that led to the end of one career opened the door to a whole new phase in my life. I now hold a PhD in anthropology and specialize in the bioarchaeological analysis of human skeletal remains. My studies have taken me to England, France, Italy, Ukraine, St. Croix, and throughout North America. I have been exposed to an entire world I would have missed had I remained a firefighter. For this, I am especially fortunate.

As for District 2, he eventually became the chief of Orlando Fire Department. I think we both got what we wanted.